To Jilli
Wishing you all the
health & happiness
Best Wishes

Dean Zoul

THRIVE!

THRIVE!

A Holistic Approach To High Performance Living

DEAN COULSON

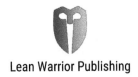

Lean Warrior Publishing

THRIVE!

First published in 2021

The author and the publisher specifically disclaim any liability, loss or risk which is incurred as a consequence, directly or indirectly, of the use and application of any contents of this work.

ISBN 978-1-7399113-0-0

CONTENTS

PART III – EMOTIONAL WELLBEING

PART IV – MENTAL FITNESS

PART V – SPIRITUAL HEALTH

I dedicate this book to my beautiful wife Joy, and my super cool son Sam. If I were to sum them up in one word that word would be...Awesome. Thank you for putting up with me and supporting me on my life's purpose.

I love you both so much x

FOREWORD

"How long have I known Dean Coulson?

Long enough to know that Thrive will be transformative to all who read it, long enough to trust his word and heed his advice and happy enough (honoured enough) to put my moniker and my validation and my reputation to this foreword and to this beautiful man.

I am excited that Dean is finally placing his earned wisdom into the eternity of ink, so that those who follow might find a guide, a map, a true path to follow, within these pages.

I saw this promise in Dean many years ago, when he was training with me in martial arts (in Coventry, England) and I invited him to teach his transformative concepts to students who had transcended physical combatives and joined me on my self sovereignty course.

These were very discerning people steeped in success, and looking only for the 'real'. Without exception they all loved Dean, they loved his presentation, and they took his teachings to heart.

I am sure that you will find concepts in this book that you have never read before, ideas that will greatly challenge your current beliefs, but, if you follow Dean's advice, THRIVE! could prove lifesaving."

Geoff Thompson

BAFTA winning Screen writer & Sunday Times Best Selling Author

PREFACE

Two life events changed the course of my journey on this brief sojourn on this spinning globe.

At the time I could not have foreseen how these events would shape my life.

The first was in my teens, watching my mam suffer with mental illness. I didn't fully understand it back then, but I knew my mam felt pain and anguish. I was frustrated that I could not help her, but at the same time angry that she wasn't always there for me. What a chemical cocktail of emotions that created for a teenager. I don't believe that now, I know she did the best she could, but when I was young it felt very real, so I vowed never to be in a position to feel that way. However in my naivety I did not fully understand why we as humans can be affected so much by our environment.

So I did what I thought was right at the time. I started to get fit. I got some weights, I started to run, I found a martial arts club and threw myself into every aspect of fitness. I was determined that I would be the fittest version of myself I could be. This determination has never left me and I have often been asked why I was so obsessed by training. This I believe is the reason.

The second was when my wife and I were told we couldn't conceive naturally. We had tried for 5 years without success. At first we didn't even consider how difficult a journey we were about to embark on; the mental and emotional turmoil we were destined to face. Day by day, month by month and nothing. We consulted the medics; we had the tests and that's when we knew.

It was my fault. Everything that could be wrong with my sperm was wrong. Volume, motility and morphology. There were very few sperm, they couldn't swim and they were all hunchbacks! The bottom line? We were told by medics 'You will NEVER be able to conceive a child naturally'.

Shell-shocked was probably what best described our state, our reality in that moment. But all was not lost. Fertility treatment was a viable option and it was offered on the NHS (National Health Service). We saw hope, a way to have what we desperately wanted. A child.

Did it go smoothly?

What do you think?

We tried twice; it failed twice.

Each time was an effort. It was an emotional strain that we were prepared to endure because we wanted to create a bundle of life to bring into this world that we would cherish, love and adore.

The first time it failed, Joy was in agony. To this day we don't know why. We had invested so much emotional energy into it. We had faith, we hoped, we had our fingers and toes crossed and it didn't happen.

We were crushed. We knew the procedure wasn't 100% effective, but with controlling all the variables and a first class fertility team we believed it would be a success. It took time to process, to understand, to feel. I will not lie. It was horrible. I felt useless. I harboured guilt that it was all my fault, a burden that I continued to carry into the second attempt months later.

I was determined to make sure that we could do everything possible to allow this process to succeed and give us what we desired.

So I started thinking about what else could help. I am stubborn and have an open mind and I refused to believe that we couldn't have our own kid.

I started researching. Back in the early 2000's the internet was still in its infancy. Information and people were nowhere near as accessible as they are now. I remember scouring Amazon for books and from internet searches came to the following conclusion. I didn't really understand health and nutrition and it was apparent that both can play a huge role in fertility.

I felt a renewed sense of optimism (this was my default setting back then, I always looked on the bright side of things). I spoke to Joy. We got out the yellow pages and found a nutritionist, called and made an appointment.

What happened at that appointment changed our lives forever.

Our eyes were opened so wide I didn't think we would ever be able to close them. Over the course of 2 hours everything was laid out. I found answers to unexplained problems I had lived with for years. Explanations to things that made so much sense, they were hidden in plain sight and yet I had had no awareness that they were even there.

We got home that evening and went to the kitchen. Everything was different. We looked in the cupboards for something to eat and found nothing. The cupboards were full and yet totally empty. We didn't eat a thing.

The food we thought was good healthy food wasn't. Most of it was processed garbage. Staples that we had grown up with were some of the primary causes of inflammation and highly likely were affecting our ability to have kids. It seemed so incredible.

I remember feeling angry, frustrated, elated and happy all at once. Frustrated and angry that Doctors had no clue about this at all, but happy and elated that we had found a different perspective; something that could help.

We were determined to do everything we could to make sure that our second fertility treatment was a success. We changed how we ate, we bought supplements and we stopped drinking alcohol.

And I kept researching. I bought books, I found studies. Not just for fertility, but for optimising every facet of health; to understand what health really meant. I became a voracious reader. I contacted nutritionists, authors of books I had found. I had so many questions.

We were confident that our second attempt at creating life via IVF would be a success.

It wasn't.

This time Joy was in so much agony we ended up in hospital all night. The Doctors didn't have a clue what was going on and just gave her painkillers. We knew deep down then that this just wasn't going to work.

If the first time was heart-breaking, the second time was devastating. We both spiralled downwards. Consumed by the denial of the one thing we both wanted. I buried my feelings because I wanted to be there for Joy. She was hurting and I hated seeing her like that.

I just did not know what to say. I had no words that would take that pain away. I remember our conversations. It put a huge strain on our relationship. It wasn't a nice time.

But we didn't give up.

We believed that we had found something. Even though IVF had not worked for us, we believed and put our faith in optimising our health and nutrition. We had frozen embryos in case we wanted to try IVF again, but our eyes had been opened.

Could 'optimising our health' give us what we wanted?

I then found a fertility nutrition book. I read it cover to cover and with my new awareness and belief around the power of nutrition we booked a consultation with the author.

We completed questionnaires, had tests and took on board their recommendations.

We were determined and hoped beyond hope this would provide the answer we had been searching for.

Three months later (the maturation time of sperm) we had decided to use our frozen embryos for a third IVF attempt and had started the procedure of hormone manipulation. A week later, Joy found out she was pregnant. She had felt something was different. She bought a pregnancy test and it came back positive. We bought another as we couldn't believe it. It told us the same... Positive! We checked with the fertility clinic to see if the drugs Joy had started taking could give a false positive. Turned out they couldn't.

She was 7 weeks pregnant. Our baby was conceived naturally!

INTRODUCTION

This book isn't about fertility or diets.

It's about health.

It's about brutal self-honesty. It's about truth and courage. It's about giving you enough information to ignite your curiosity.

For you to wake up from your slumber and start THRIVING!

You don't have time to just 'survive' in your lifetime, there is so much more waiting for you. Don't settle for second best. Forget waiting for tomorrow (for it never comes), forget waiting for Monday, next week, next month, next year!

Your time to thrive is now.

Before you start reading this book, I want you to stop.

I want you to ask yourself, "What do I want out of it?"

If you are after another quick fix to put your life on track then this ain't it.

That is what puts you on a merry-go-round. You condition your brain to look for failure. You buy into those beliefs and you will ALWAYS go out of your way to prove your unconscious beliefs true. Even if consciously you say you want to change, deep down there will be incongruence, your wants will be out of alignment with your beliefs and willpower will never cut it long term.

Don't believe me?

There are so many times I can remember when I have tried to force through change and been met with massive resistance.

Willpower is good to get you out of the blocks, but it will not get you to your final destination. Most of the time, we use willpower to endure something for a period of time, that we don't like or want to do. How will that ever serve you?

But dig a little deeper; go beyond your surface level wants and you ask yourself WHY that is important to you. If you are brave and really challenge those reasons and start feeling into your emotions, you will find your truth. Maybe you want to lose weight, or tone yourself up, get a new job or feel loved.

Is it easy?

In a word, no. It is one of the most challenging journeys you can ever embark upon, finding out who you are and why you are on this spinning globe.

Is it worth it?

Absolutely!

When you start contracting and start challenging the stories, reasons and excuses you hold that stop you having the life that you want. When you remove people, possessions and things that deep down you know no longer serve you, you create space for expansion for what sets your soul on fire, what you truly desire and what makes your heart sing.

It's in there believe me. I know because I have felt it, I have experienced it and after every contraction and expansion I have felt power; an energy surge, a feeling that anything is possible. My life being in my control, that feeling that I can achieve anything. Once I allowed myself to see, to have the awareness, it opened the door to see what else was possible.

So I ask you. What do you truly want? What is it that is holding you back? What has you anchored in your past? What beliefs do you hold keeping you stuck?

I invite you to suspend those beliefs for now, to consider ALL possibilities. Open your mind to the belief that you can thrive in your life. The evidence is all around, people are doing it. There are no unfair advantages, just hard work and an open mind. By rolling up your sleeves and facing your truth you can have it too.

But make no mistake, if all your thinking is anchoring you in the past then that's where you will stay. Until you cut that baggage loose, until you surrender to the bigger picture and have the faith that you can create the life you want, you will always fall short.

Is that what you really want?

Ask yourself right now and see what comes back to you.

Life is fraught with challenges. Most of us have a certain world view based on our conditioning, beliefs and past experiences.

Unbeknown to you, your 'comfort zone' is preventing you from seeing what is really possible.

Even as I write 'comfort zone' I laugh, as it is just another narrative, another label to attach meaning to and hide behind. Another way to put barriers in front of you, another reason or excuse...

If you allow it to be.

You can hide behind bravado to misdirect others about how you are feeling, but you can never fool yourself. YOU KNOW. In those quiet moments, when your guard is down (and I know all about dropping my guard), you feel that discomfort. You hear the voices in your head, the sub-personalities vying for your attention. Those masks you put in place to fit in with other people's lives. But what about your life? Is it that meaningless that you dismiss it out of hand just so others might like you?

I have a radical idea, how about liking yourself first?

Scratch that, how about learning to love yourself first?

Realise that on this planet, your life matters; **you matter**. You do not have to fit in with another person's ideals to be enough. You are enough right now.

Are you here to make up the numbers?

Or are you here to step up and make a difference?

You get to choose.

YOU GET TO THRIVE!

The first step is to expand your awareness.

Everything starts with awareness. Awareness precedes change. How can we change anything if we are not aware of what else is possible?

Immediately after that, is having an open mind. Why? Because your beliefs, shadows, sub-personalities will fight for survival. They with cajole you and vie for your attention to stop you from changing.

Self-protection starts with the self. You get to defend yourself against your inner bully, the stories, scripts and conditioning keeping you imprisoned. The big scary three dimensional monster we create in our minds to prevent us having everything we ever wanted.

But when we challenge, when we stop running, when we turn around and face that monster with love, that three dimensional monster becomes a two dimensional cartoon. It is illusory. Everything we have ever wanted lies just beyond it.

THRIVE! will lead you to that place. Just get to open the door and have the courage to step through.

Ready?

PART I - IT'S ALL YOUR FAULT

| 1 |

Where Have All the Warriors Gone?

I remember a time when people lived a challenging and purposeful existence and were more vibrant and passionate for it.

Today I see a world full of whiners, moaners and whingers, who have completely lost track of who they really are. They don't know how to break a sweat or know how to handle discomfort anymore. They don't know how to protect themselves from themselves, never mind protect their loved ones. They run to the pub, the fridge or the doctor to hide, to sedate their mundane existence instead of facing up to the discomfort of life and taking the lessons head on.

Life is for living, for thriving and yet I see a planet shrouded in fear, people cowering and hiding, simply existing day to day trying to survive.

We are not here for that!

We are here to take control of our lives in any moment, to face whatever stands before us and simply ask "What is the worst thing that could happen by doing this?"

Fear can terrorise us if we allow it.

Read that again "if we allow it".

Nothing can happen to you unless you *allow it to.*

Once you understand this, you will realise that no one can 'make you' do anything or feel a certain way. Only you can do that. That's when you can take back the power you give away to others. You get to recognise what is resonating inside you when people or situations trigger you and the actions you must take to avoid or attack what makes you uncomfortable.

So what do you fear? What are you hiding from?

What paralyses you and prevents you from having everything in your life that you desire?

Where does the discomfort come from?

Your imagination.

We are fuelled by stories that we have chosen to believe; the opinions of others who have no place shaping our world based on their own shortcomings and insecurities.

Fuelled by the fear that has enveloped you because of it, that you are not good enough, that you are not worth it, that you will be judged and ridiculed if you don't "toe the line".

To hell with that!

Culture, conditioning and societal norms would have you act and behave in a certain way to 'fit in'. Indeed your brain works in such a way that you are "hardwired" to be part of a group to promote survival of the species.

But why do we need to conform to the majority?

The answer is you don't, you are conditioned to fear change, but other than actual physical danger, fear is an illusion that you create.

Embrace Your Fears

Discomfort is essential for you to grow. It is to be embraced, not feared. It is there to test you, to see how much you want to change, to test the fabric of your existence in this world. It is there to see how certain you are that the path you are on is the right one.

It will call you out. It will challenge you. It will ask "Who are you to do that?"

And if you are not clear, if you lack certainty, if you do not know, then it can and often will consume you. Living in a state of self-doubt, lacking confidence and looking for permission on how to live your life instead of drawing a line and shouting…

"I know who I am and what I believe. I know what my values are!"

Where is Our Hardiness?

So what is happening to the human race? The ever expanding waistlines and home comforts are making humans soft. We are caught up in the blame culture. We are being made soft by everything around us.

The word 'warrior' literally translates to "the bravery to face oneself."

- Are you brave enough to face your own fears?
- Are you ready to be brutally honest with yourself?
- Are you ready to challenge EVERY story you hold dear that does NOT serve you?
- Are you ready to change the belief you have around that story?

- Are you ready to fully feel the discomfort and let it go?

The vitality from expressing your inner warrior brings about confidence and congruence that permeates every aspect of your life. You just have to let it out.

Isn't it time to express yourself?

We live increasingly sedentary lives when we were designed for much more. We inhabit bodies that are built to move and yet they have become a soft outer shell. The body needs demanding work to stay healthy; our minds need challenge and purpose.

Our ancestry is still inside us; we are still warriors within. This must be reclaimed and expressed, not hidden and repressed.

Isn't it time to explore what you believe, what you stand for and what you stand against?

Isn't it time to take time to define what your values are and what they mean to you?

I for one have had enough. We exist for more than this. We are here to thrive not to survive!

Transformation is typically defined as a physical appearance being drastically changed, for the better. But I see it as much more than that. I see transformation as your whole life experience, every fabric of your being.

Every facet of your life challenged and turned on its head.

Optimising your health, exploring each of the four areas of the health paradigm (physical, mental, emotional and spiritual) to see how they can be improved and highlight what is standing in your way for you to challenge and optimise.

Find out your 'why', your purpose for being on this mortal coil.

Doing so will allow you to move forwards with purpose and energy you never thought possible.

That is the purpose of this book. To wake you up from your slumber. To give you an awareness of what is possible. To allow you to challenge where you are in your life right now and question every thought and belief. To see whether you truly are living a thriving life or whether you have been fooled into believing you are living your life, when in fact, it was someone else's wishes.

It's time to step up. Find your essence, your true, authentic self through brutal introspection and to face your adversity. Find the courage to face down your stories and beliefs, fuelled by your imagination and create a new reality, one that serves you.

Now is the time...

To take back control, embrace extreme ownership over the self.

To live a purposeful life and gain self-sovereignty over the self.

For freedom, fulfilment and true power.

To exercise your true will and powerful imagination!

And create a life you desire... for you.

A life to THRIVE!

| 2 |

Take Your Power Back

So how do you do it?

Three things…

Acute **awareness**!

Radical **responsibility**!

Awesome **action**!

I could have just written awareness, responsibility and action, but I wanted to big them up a bit ;-)

Awareness

The first step is always awareness. I see so many people switched off, oblivious to their surroundings, code white. How often do you see people on the street in their own little worlds? Maybe you have spent time there yourself?

When I teach physical self-protection, I always start with awareness. Having awareness prevents you from entering situations that could be physically unsafe. If you have awareness then you become a hard target.

Metaphysically it is the same. Self-protection always begins with the self, defending yourself against your inner bully. That voice in your head trying to keep you down and hold you back (and it will if you let it).

To change something you first have to have an awareness of it. Awareness precedes change after all.

Otherwise you will continue in the humdrum of life getting what you always got.

Do you think that by behaving is such a way will allow you to thrive?

Having awareness is like waking up, tuning into something for the first time.

See the world, YOUR world through different eyes.

This is empowering. In that moment you can make a choice to take responsibility.

Responsibility

Understanding that everything you have thought said and done up to this point is your fault. You are to blame. If that stings a bit, then good. If you are reacting then you get to make a choice, to keep blaming and giving your personal power away or to accept responsibility. Only then can you do something about your current situation and choose differently.

How empowering is that?

Action

Simply choose to begin. Take action out of faith, what feels good, what your intuition says, not your head. Intuition is about feeling NOT thinking. Isn't thinking what got you here in the first place? Removing the internal self-limiting emotions allows you to move forward without the brakes on.

Does it feel scary?

Yes it does. There will be resistance. Your inner bully will not let go without a metaphorical fight. Years of conditioning can weigh heavy, but if you know how to let things go and be brave you can have a thriving life!

So step forward you must, to act in spite of the fear you feel, with courage and an understanding that we are not in danger, not really. However, by imagining and creating big scary monsters, those beliefs that keep us cowering in fear and running for cover, we remain stuck.

So by facing your fears, you expose your darkness to the light, fears to knowledge and courage.

Triumph over adversity

We all have crosses to bear. We all have first world problems. It is how we deal with them that defines who we are; whether you live from a victor state or a victim state; whether you are brave and stand up as your truest version of yourself in spite of how you feel, or you allow past beliefs to dictate how you think, what you say and how you act.

Come to terms with the value you create in this world by standing up and giving it the benefit of your wisdom. Do not rob the world of that.

In those moments of stillness, of clarity, when the stars align, we muster the courage to keep going, to keep challenging the stories, to accept the pain we feel and sit with it, feel it, observe it and ultimately let it go.

It just isn't that easy.

When we truly wake up and become self-aware, we become truth seekers. In the cold light of day we stand alone as we always have; standing in front of a mirror and asking the searching questions; having brutal self-honesty by facing every fear you have buried deep. Finding the truest version of yourself takes courage, tenacity and discipline.

That's when you get to ask.

Do I want to survive or thrive?

| 3 |

Happiness is a Choice

I have had conversations with so many people about choice. I have been told by many that they had no choice or there isn't a choice. Even I have said this in the past. But here's the thing…

You always have a choice.

It's just that sometimes it feels too uncomfortable or painful and when it feels painful you move away from it. Your brain wants you to feel safe all of the time and so will take the steps to ensure you are (even to the detriment of your health).

Humans often use every reason they can to justify wanting something; the next fad or diet, new house, car, holiday, new job, new baby, partner, new clothes, or just to be happy and fulfilled.

But the answer is never there, so they keep looking.

And that's the problem; searching outside of oneself.

You are looking externally for your happiness, you keep searching and searching, but always come up short.

But what if you just stopped?

What if you just realised that happiness is not without, but within?

What if you just decided to be happy and realise that it has been your choice all along?

What if you were just too scared to just stop and face the truth that it is a choice?

So just decide to be happy.

"In the end, we only regret the chances we didn't take"

- LEWIS CARROLL

The path to happiness starts with removing what makes you unhappy. What drains your energy? What feels heavy? What are you doing that you hate? Who do you put up with? What thoughts are you entertaining that do not serve you?

Stop dragging things around with you that don't light you up.

Simple strategies are rarely easy. They usually trigger all kinds of emotions and yet they are the route to true happiness.

Start by letting go of things that fill you with dread and start discovering what fills your heart with joy, introducing them into your life.

Be brutal about protecting your time and energy, only doing the non-negotiables; those impeccable agreements you made with yourself (in blood) to raise your standards that you DO NOT compromise on. These are the things that set your soul on fire and make your heart sing.

What does that look like for you? I mean REALLY look like?

Have you ever just stopped and asked yourself this question?

Have you looked at everything you are doing right now and asked, "Does this make me happy?"

If it is not making you happy, why are you doing it?

Look around and realise YOUR happiness must come first. There are no prerequisites, no conditions. Happiness will not be found in material objects; there is no quick fix. Happiness is remembering who you are and why you are here; a state of peace, harmony and bliss.

You can choose to start being happy, today, now!

BE happy by doing the things that give you happiness (and only those things)!

Now I know some of you, you might get triggered by what I am saying, you might feel annoyed. That is good that is a perfect place to start.

If you are not prepared to challenge and question every story you believe to be true about why you are not happy, sit with the uncomfortable sensations they create that you usually avoid and fully feel them and let them go, you will remain stuck.

The power is in you to transform yourself. It comes from the realisation that creating the happiness you crave, starts with a choice.

It is not about **HAVE – DO - BE**

Having things and doing things to be who you are, does not lead to happiness.

Start with being 'you'. Remove the mask you wear in order to fit in and have the courage to be yourself.

BE – DO - HAVE

First of all, who are you? How can you be happy? Where will you live? Who will you spend your time with? How will you spend your day? What is your purpose? Ask yourself those questions. Be brutally honest with your answers. What is that ideal day you dare to dream about?

Darkness and light

I don't pretend to know how your life has been, but I do know that you can uncover the happiness you crave.

I just want to be clear. Happiness is an emotion and as with any emotion it has energy attached to it.

E-Motion… Energy in Motion after all.

Energy is finite and emotions are transient and so we get to protect that energy and be aware of how we are feeling.

Recognise, that there are times when life just beats you and that is ok. There is nothing wrong with you. Even 'successful' people have their low moods and 'down' moments. Use them as an alarm, to alert you that something needs to change. This shows you what you are focusing on right now. Maybe it's an old script or story you get to challenge; maybe it's an expectation you are trying to live up to or even a situation that is triggering something in you.

Allow yourself to fully feel the sensation. Low moods or triggers often appear to highlight something to address or to let go of. Whatever thoughts you might be having observe them. You are not your thoughts. The more you face this the more you can become a master of your emotions.

That way you can engineer how often you feel happiness.

You must know darkness to truly understand light. They form a dichotomy, a contrast. You cannot truly know one without experiencing the other. There are times when you might feel the world is against you and you just want to crawl back under the duvet. In reality though it is a shift, a gift giving you the feedback to realise what to look at next.

But what is happiness?

I had to dig deep to really understand it. It's easy to get happiness mixed up with pleasure. Happiness is driven from within; an appreciation of all that you have and not having to prove anything to anyone or live up to others ideals or expectations of others. Pleasure is often a fleeting gratification triggered by some external event or need; driven by the hormone dopamine (also known as the seeking hormone), which soon fades requiring another fix.

What if happiness is defined by creating something meaningful for you; having a true appreciation for what you already have and defining meaning, why you are here?

What are you committing to?

You always get what you commit to. Look around. Are you happy with your life right now? No? Then look deeper at why your current commitments are more important to you than the happiness you crave. We often attach emotions to situations that are too painful to face and so we unknowingly create stories and beliefs to take us away from that pain.

You will always find the time, energy and focus for things that are truly important to you. So what are you making important? If you say you want happiness but the actions you take are making you unhappy, you are out of alignment.

What you say you want consciously is in conflict with what you truly believe unconsciously and you will ALWAYS go out of your way to prove your beliefs are true. That's when you challenge those beliefs, allowing yourself to fully feel anything that makes you uncomfortable. That is the key to letting go of what makes you unhappy.

Realise this...

Each day is a gift and not a given right. It is too easy to take things for granted. We live in expectation that we will open our eyes each day instead of being grateful that we do. Life is finite and we literally do not know how long we have. Don't waste a single moment. Do not take anything for granted in your life, appreciate everything you have.

Change your perspective; be open to a different point of view.

It is so easy to get caught up in your own first world problems. That's when you get to stop, breathe and step back. Take that 30,000 foot view to create a different perspective, you might just see how fruitless the drama you create really is.

No matter who you are, you can BE who you want to be; you can DO what you want to do!

Do not stand in your own way. Time ticks on regardless whatever you choose to do. No matter how much you may want to you cannot rewind a moment in your life, time is never on your side.

So ask yourself this right now...

"If today was my last day, what would I do?"

Would you decide, today, to be happy?

Would you let go of the things you are harbouring, the envy, jealousy, grudges? Would you forgive others? Would you forgive yourself?

Would you allow yourself to do what you want, what you love, with whom you love?

Would you let go of the past (what makes you unhappy)?

Choose today to BE that day.

Take your first step towards your happiness.

Imagine! What would that be like?

Stop reading right now, take out a note pad and pen and write down how YOUR perfect day would look for you. Be selfish. How would you be feeling? Where would you be living? What would you be doing? Who would you be with?

START, THERE, NOW!

| 4 |

The Health Paradigm

I believe we are synergistic beings. I see four elements of true health that intertwine and if we are brave, if we dare to look at what is possible, will take us from just 'surviving' day to day to 'thriving'.

But what does thrive mean?

To thrive is to grow and develop vigorously; to flourish, be successful in our endeavours and feel happy and fulfilled.

The context of this book is to optimise the four elements of your health; to actively look to improve each area and raise your standards and no longer accept mediocrity.

After all, that is what we are here to do; to live life to the full. Unfortunately I see few doing so. I see so many stuck in the matrix (remember neo?); so many unwilling or unable to break free. The truth is hidden in plain sight; it is right there in front of you if you are courageous and willing to look.

It all starts with awareness, that moment of clarity where everything makes sense, something feels different, you are different, seeing things with new vision. It may even trigger people, when we have moments of clarity and respond differently in our lives, to become mirrors for others, often for those closest to us. We reflect in others what they don't want to see. Quite often they try and pull you back down to their level to ease their discomfort.

"It's easier to pull someone out of a tree than to make the effort to climb up beside them."

Few having that awareness, a knowing deep down there is something more to life; that uneasy feeling that is difficult to explain. It is a gnawing inside the pit of your stomach that won't go away no matter what you do to distract yourself; it can feel incongruous.

I know when I found my awareness, a realisation of what my purpose was and why I am here on this spinning globe, everything changed. I sent a ripple out from my epicentre that affected everything single thing around me. Some friends fell away never to be seen again. Some felt aggrieved or uncomfortable. Some tried to challenge me and even belittle me to get me to be the old version of myself. Maybe you have felt that, however fleetingly. Sometimes it just feels too scary to contemplate, other times it feels so exciting.

There are no absolutes in life and yet; those closed minded to all possibilities will defend their path and that is fine. They are just not ready, unable or unwilling to see a different path. Their heart closed down due to feelings of fear, shame or guilt.

But it's not about one path, one way. I believe there is always a way, there is always a solution, some path to follow, often the path less travelled.

It is not about either/or, one or the other. It's about embracing AND, the two together. Why does their have to be sacrifice when we can have it all?

To thrive, we get to be brave. We get to let go; we get to face down every obstacle; we get to nourish ourselves and accept who we are.

Who says that we have to compromise?

Who says that we cannot live life to the full?

I believe we can have it all.

Is it easy? No!

Is it challenging? Absolutely!

But that doesn't make it impossible.

You get to choose to raise your standards.

You get to remove the non-essentials.

You get create time for the non-negotiables, those impeccable agreements you can make for yourself that you live your life by, to thrive!

You have the time to address all 4 elements of health; physical, mental, emotional and spiritual.

This book will address each one and give you an awareness to investigate further; to look past the common narrative; to redefine what normal means to you; to look past societal moors and cultural bias. You will challenge the stories you currently believe.

Just because someone says it's true, doesn't mean it is. So challenge everything, even what I am saying.

Open Pandora's Box; open your eyes to what is possible. See past what you are fed day in day out.

You have that choice. It's what you do with that choice that counts.

Whether you choose to blame or validate why you are stuck or whether you become curious and accept responsibility and take your power back over your life.

You get to choose.

Oh and for those who think there isn't a choice?

Even not choosing is choosing.

| 5 |

What is Health Anyway?

Before my 'awakening', seeing health as I do now, I believed what I was told, without question. In fact, it didn't even occur to me to challenge what the word 'health' meant, which foods nourished and which were, let's say, 'less than ideal'. I just followed the common narrative fed to me by the government, those 'in charge' and media advertising. I blindly accepted that whatever food supermarkets sold, must be ok to eat and eat it I did.

But when my wife and I were told we couldn't have kids I began to have doubts about the health information I had believed, no longer accepting it as 'my truth'. I didn't get the concept of unexplained infertility. I didn't accept that 'a low sperm count' was something that could not be addressed. I believed there had to be another way. I started to wonder what could be stopping us when it seemed so easy for everyone else. That's when I started to look for solutions and explored what 'health' really meant.

Everyone I have come across since I started helping people to 'thrive' believes that they are healthy.

But here's the rub. Most people are not healthy. They have an idea fed to them (pun intended) without challenging it. That is my experience having worked with hundreds of people.

You may feel the same. The word 'health' is thrown around way too easily. Everyone has their own definition, mostly from sources that were trusted and accepted without question.

There are so many myths that perpetuate regarding what health actually is, mostly from companies whose vested interest is in their profits and NOT your health. They will tell you what you want to hear so they can make a fast buck. Too many people are willing to accept aches and pains or not 'feeling right' as something that is age-related. The only thing that comes close to that is the amount of time that you have been willing to endure it; it has nothing to do with getting old.

Health is a state of being.

It's not about eating "low fat" dietary products or having energy drinks touted as "essential to get through each day".

There is a world of confusion regarding health and wellbeing. Supermarkets, food manufacturers, even the government, manipulate you and feed your insecurities about who you are, how you look, what you think you need for health, how you feel and what you fear.

We are so conditioned to follow the next fad or quick fix; the majority jumping from one thing to the next without any thought about why.

But why do you need it?

It seems that we have lost the ability to trust our own intuition, preferring to accept the opinions and advice of complete strangers, without question.

During the course of my research, I discovered that most people have no idea what they should be eating. Does that sound like you?

If so, you have allowed someone else to take responsibility for what you eat, so you don't have to. That means it isn't "your fault" if you put on weight or have no energy, it is someone else's.

How disempowering!

Everyone recognises 'healthy foods' and everyone knows broccoli is better than chocolate or water is better than fizzy drinks. It's the mindless brain washing that confuses people.

As a health/transformation coach I come across a myriad of people, each one believing they are healthy and this may well be true. However, there are others who have a different view.

Some think moderation is key; some think living in solitude, living 100% clean and living off the land without external influence is health. Others still have no idea what health is or simply don't care, usually to their detriment.

"If you don't make time for your health, at some point you WILL make time for illness."

There are companies who are only interested in manipulating your choice of product to take your hard-earned money.

Everyone has their own idea or definition of health and there have been endless discussions about what contributes to health and how to improve it.

So let's look at my definition of 'health' and see what you think.

What is my Definition of Health?

Can we really define health as a whole or is it a unique experience?

One dictionary defines health as "the state of being free from illness or injury".

But health isn't just about surviving as is suggested by the definition above. I think it is way more, as you may have guessed by now I think it's about THRIVING!

The world health organisation defines health differently

"Health is a state of complete physical, mental and social well-being and not merely the absence of disease or infirmity."

This is more in line with what I believe to be true, so let's delve deeper.

In my opinion, the word 'health' means so much more than what people may realise.

Enter Nutrition

I was searching for a solution to my infertility.

Understanding and studying what nourishes the body was my starting point. I had a goal to reverse infertility and so I started reading about and studying nutrition. I contacted nutritionists. In fact I dug out the yellow pages (well it was the early 2000's and the advent of social media was just a sparkle in someone's eye and the internet was in its infancy), found a nutritionist and made an appointment for my wife and I to go. What an eye opener! We were informed that there was a solution, something could be done. A glimmer of hope!

I learned that everything we ingest has a major impact on our health. We needed to address deficiencies and remove what was toxic for the body. Over time, this would have a major impact on how healthy our bodies could be. But it was not just about the food; it was about the chemicals used in crop spraying, the contents of our water supply, and what we cook with etc.

Next, I sought out nutritionists who were experts in infertility. As a result our son was born naturally in 2004.

This was all down to having a better understanding of what health means and how to nourish the body to thrive. And yes, nutrition is THAT powerful!

Now I see nutrition as PART of health, not all of it. There is so much more to it that than people realise. Nutrition is still a vital part and it is very powerful; it has the power to gift life, even in the most difficult of circumstances.

It is not just what you eat (or more appropriately ingest) it is about how well you digest your food to get the nutrients you need. It is about proper hydration, breathing correctly, emotional balance, getting enough sleep, rest and recovery, how you are handling stress, how you move as well as what you let into your head and heart.

THEY ALL PLAY A PART!

Health is not just a one trick pony, it is multifaceted. It is all about finding a balance in all areas of your life, not just one or two.

It is about having all the bases covered and being VERY truthful about where you are and what has to improve to tap into your vast power and becoming the pinnacle of health.

How Do You Define Health?

What health means differs for many people.

Firstly, some simply believe that you are healthy because you are not sick, there is no disease present, well not one defined by the medical profession.

But health is so much more than not having a disease. You can be disease free and live a sub life; a life devoid of laughter, passion, fun, love, energy and vitality (to name just a few).

You can have your physical health, eat well and rest, but have poor relationships and be unhelpful and feel unfulfilled.

Or you can have the opposite, being of poor health and diet, poor sleep but have an enriched life through deep connections with others, having fun and making a difference to other people's lives.

Ideally we are looking to encompass the best of all these examples and yet, few people strive for it.

So Is Health Really Just the Absence of Disease?

I don't believe it is.

It is not about focusing on what you don't have (disease), but what you do have. Health is about living a full life; having the energy to accomplish anything; having the resilience to face any challenge; allowing yourself to grow and become all that you can be.

Disease just does not come into it. To claim you are healthy because you are not sick is robbing you of your life and vitality, of what is REALLY possible. There are other things at play that can prevent you from living a full healthy life without being diagnosed with some condition.

"The microbe is nothing; the terrain is everything."

– CLAUDE BERNARD

Louis Pasteur (who invented pasteurisation) is the godfather of medicine, on which today's modern medicine is based. He noted that germs were the source of viruses and disease and his "germ theory" is what is used today in modern medicine.

He based his whole theory on the prevention of germs and disagreed with the above quote made by his contemporary Claude Bernard until his deathbed. Louis Pasteur then admitted that the above statement was actually true, that when a body is in homeostasis or balance and in strong health with a strong immune system it can look after itself and kill the germs that lead to viruses and diseases.

But Pasteur's initial work on germ theory had already become most prevalent, and still is, which is why Doctors try and kill all germs with drugs and keep hospitals sterile. Thankfully, more information is coming to the forefront all the time about cellular health, healthy gut flora, probiotic foods, strengthening immunity, and preventing disease holistically.

Our stomachs are living ecosystems full of bacteria which sustain our lives. Healthy colonies of good bacteria help protect us from bad bacteria, and without the good gut flora we have little defence. True, people with severely weakened immune systems have to be careful not contract pathogenic germs, but the normal ideal is to have a strong immune system that wards off pathogens that we come in contact with every day, without needing to hide from them.

It just seems that so many people have lost the ability to trust themselves; to trust what their body is capable of if they look after it. We must understand that we have been on this planet for millennia and despite everything humans have been exposed to we are still here. Fear permeates in the lives of so many that they stop trusting how amazing they are and can be, especially when you put your health first.

Is Perfect Health Possible?

Health and what it means is so diverse that maintaining a true balance of everything that contributes to it can be challenge... but NOT impossible.

I believe you have to look at all areas of your life separately, to see whether you have your bases covered. If not, you must decide how you can upgrade and optimise each area.

Balance – Your relationship with yourself, your family and your friends. Being honest and transparent, not buying into gossip or lies, the sensationalism that people seem to thrive on these days. Check where your attention is, do you allow yourself to be affected by adulation or criticism? You don't need validation or permission to live your life. You get to control how you feel by being in balance with how you think and feel. Strive to tell the truth, starting with what you tell yourself. This is so easily dismissed. To avoid judgement from others we take to wearing (metaphorical) masks and live lives that others want us to live and not what we were placed on this earth for. Be fully immersed in your connections with others, especially those closest to you, do not be distracted and maintain total focus.

Body – What you eat/drink and moving with purpose. Everything to give yourself the best performing body you can with a strong immune system to ward off everyday bugs and viruses. Humans were built to move, not sit all day on our backsides. You inhabit an amazing vehicle, the only one you own in fact. You get to look after it and by doing so it will allow you to experience amazing things.

Remember that nutrition can give life, it is that powerful. Never neglect it. Assess yours. What stories do you tell yourself as to why you cannot give something up that doesn't serve you? Challenge any addictive behaviours, almost always driven by something deeper. Challenge your beliefs, are you eating like an adult or a child?

Being – What you do to BE yourself; to put yourself first; to attain your own happiness and fulfilment. To allow yourself time to practise being in the present moment, to let go of the past and stop thinking about the future. This may sound selfish but if you are not 100% healthy, physically, emotionally, mentally and spiritually then how can you give 100% to your partner or kids?

If you are run ragged by putting yourself down the pecking order, if you are running at 50% or less because you put yourself last, how can you ever give anymore to others? Allow yourself the time to recharge those batteries so you can help others more effectively, never neglect yourself or think you are not worth it.

Meditation, practising mindfulness, spiritual study, journaling, affirmations and visualisations can have a massive impact on your health and help you focus and believe in who you are. Be consistent, be persistent, be frequent. Make a commitment to yourself to optimise your health.

Holding onto or suppressing negative emotions can often manifest itself into all manner of things including diseases and is well proven. Your power is in your vulnerability, allow yourself the courage to step up and be yourself.

Business – YOUR business. What you were put on this earth for. Your passion, your purpose. Identifying who you are and who you are going to show up in the world as. I believe everyone is born with a purpose, but few have the awareness or courage to step out of the shadows. Are you aligned with who you are meant to be?

Do you know what sets your soul on fire and your heart sing? Are you providing your knowledge and your uniqueness to the world or are you hiding it away? Become very clear on your value and how to share it with the world and then take the first step. Once you have that awareness (often hidden in plain sight) and realise why you are here, only you can stop yourself from moving forward. Only you can look at the stories and past conditioning and challenge the truth of it and how you can transform yourself, however I have found that a guide or teacher will show up when you are ready. I have experienced that many times in my life.

Buzz – What is life without a bit of fun? Making sure there is room every day to smile, laugh and have fun. There is not one piece of evidence I have found that says we have to live life so seriously and yet how often do you get caught up in that very thing. Make time laugh every day. It completely changes your state and raises your energy.

Remember…

If you are out of balance or out of alignment in one area, all other areas are affected too. To expand, first you have to contract. You have to shed the superfluous, get rid of the unnecessary, minimise the excess and remove the redundant so you are left with the essence of your being, no ostentation. Only then you can create the space in which to expand. Address the unhealthy areas in your life and change them.

Does it feel scary? Yes absolutely, but there is no growth in comfort. When you have the courage to be vulnerable, what you thought was your greatest weakness reveals itself to be your greatest strength.

BE Selfish!

So many people associate the word 'selfish' with negativity. But is it? I get the dictionary term, however selfishness doesn't have to be a bad thing. It can be good to be a little selfish to take care of your emotional, mental, spiritual and physical well-being. Many people who focus entirely on give, give, give end up overwhelmed, fatigued, and stressed even depressed.

So is creating time for yourself selfish?

I would argue not; everyone needs their own space to breathe and let off some steam, to contemplate and reenergise.

Should you be selfish in attaining your health?

One word... YES!

It is difficult to give 100% to other areas of your life such as family and friendships when you are not 100% yourself.

If you have ever been on an aeroplane, you are told at the start of every flight that in the case of an emergency you must fit your own oxygen mask first, before attempting to help others; for very good reason as I am sure you'll agree... you cannot help anyone else before you help yourself.

This applies to your life too.

Your health is much more than not having an illness. It is about LIVING and cutting the things loose that stop you from doing achieving a full life, being ALL that you can be. It is about being brutally honest and finding the truth to YOUR happiness and your purpose for living.

Health is about having good eating habits and exercising. It is increasing real connections to the people who matter the most to you and being present, without distraction. It is about being outside in nature as much as possible and also releasing internal self-limiting emotions and exploring who you really are.

You have more power than you can possible imagine.

What you may not realise is that having your health gives you that power.

BE Mindful, live your dreams, live your life, live your purpose and (most importantly) attain your health, when you do you will THRIVE!

| 6 |

Am I Safe?

As you go through the chapters of this book you will begin to notice a common theme. One of the secrets to thriving is to make sure you feel safe and that your brain is constantly checking your body and environment. Feeling unsafe has a huge impact on your health and your ability to thrive.

It may sound ludicrous in this modern world to ask yourself the question, "Do I feel Safe?" After all, statistically, the world is safer than it has ever been. But what about your world?

Safety comes after survival in your foundational human needs. Once your survival needs are met, (air, water, food, warmth, shelter, movement), you then look to ask the question, "Am I safe?"

Of course on the surface you think of course I am! There are no sabre tooth tigers chasing you around these days. I get it.

However I am not referring to whether your external world is safe. I am talking about your inner world. Your brain is the ultimate survival machine.

Your brain constantly checks on your safety.

That could be to see if you are physically able to move. You may have been in physical pain before. Maybe you consulted a chiropractor who has adjusted you, only for the pain to return. Why do you think that is?

I will tell you...

From a movement perspective, your brain will make sure that you are able to escape (metaphorical) danger, even if that means you are in pain. Movement might be impaired, but your body will do whatever is necessary to allow you to keep moving, even changing your movement dynamics to feel stable (or safe).

Have you really understood the cause of your pain?

If your movement is unsafe, your body will tighten muscles and lock joints down to create stability as a protection against potential injury (in case you fall and injure yourself). This can cause dysfunctional movement patterns, which, unless addressed, can lead to pain in the future.

Addressing the symptoms without establishing the underlying cause can inadvertently destabilise your body, deeming it unsafe and overriding the effects of your treatment.

Over time if these underlying imbalances are not addressed, you can end up in chronic pain. Barring any trauma, we should normally move and function without pain. Alas that isn't always the case.

So if you have recurring pain or injuries, make sure you find a physical therapist who uses any symptoms to look deeper to investigate the real cause (check out the resources page for details of who to see for an integrative approach to physical therapy). They work with the body to identify the actual cause of your pain.

Something else to consider...

When dealing with mental turmoil or emotional repression, your brain, sensing that you are unsafe, may actually lockdown or restrict physical movement. Research shows that physical pain can come from repressed or blocked emotions. It is your body's way of telling you that something needs to be addressed. Ignoring the symptoms can cause them to worsen over time until you have no option but to address them.

If you are in mental anguish, are you engaging in your thoughts, especially the thoughts that do not serve you? Are you creating a world of hell inside your mind sponsored by fear? Are you creating mind forged manacles to keep you shackled to a reality that no longer serves you?

These thoughts will trigger your fight or flight response, preparing your body to run or fight to survive. Your brain cannot differentiate what is real or imagined and you can find yourself creating a world of pain where your thoughts can affect you physically.

If you are suppressing your emotions, every time you're fight or flight response is triggered how do you react? Do you respond logically, in a calm manner or do you react and do what you programmed your brain to do when feeling stressed to protect you from emotional overwhelm, repressing emotions you haven't dealt with? Burying it, ignoring it or distracting yourself because it feels too painful to express?

Research now shows that radical acceptance of all of our emotions, even the ones we feel are difficult such as pain, loss, grief and regret, is the cornerstone to emotional resilience, thriving and true, authentic happiness.

Also consider your language; your use of words. We attach our own meanings to words depending on our current world view (our outlook on life) without any consideration as to whether they are true. This can trigger some form of drama that could easily have been avoided.

Words are essential. We use quick and easy labels to describe our own feelings without giving thought to their true meaning. For example, there is a difference between stress and disappointment. By looking deeper at our emotions we are able to more accurately discern the cause of our feelings. What is the emotion telling you? What does your heart want you to recognise and listen to?

Curiosity, compassion and the ability to take the courage to face your personal adversity is the key to lowering your stress response and allow your brain to feel safe once again, so you can take back control.

PART II – PHYSICAL HEALTH

| 7 |

Moving With Purpose.

I am not about to give you a million ways to workout. Although I have worked in the fitness industry for a number of years, coaching many people to optimise their movement, fitness and performance, this is not what this book is about.

This book is about thriving in all elements of health and that includes, not only moving with purpose, but moving pain free; bringing awareness to what I see as the most beneficial way for you guys to move.

To do that I will share with you why I believe all movement is not 'created equal' and just because something works for one person, doesn't mean it will be good for you.

Simply typing 'exercise' into google, or other internet search engine of your choice, will produce more workouts than you could ever need.

However, there is still a right way and a wrong way to move... for you personally. It's not about getting beasted or exercising to exhaustion (anyone can do that), it's about understanding your body and training intelligently for maximum effect.

By looking at the principles of movement, it's up to you to choose which method you use to adopt that principle.

You see principles never alter, only the methods of applying those principles. The primary movement patterns of humans don't change. They will always be push, pull, squat, lunge, hinge and rotate. It's how you apply these movements in a safe and effective way for YOUR body.

Yes I said YOUR body.

Just because you can, doesn't mean you should.

Remember the question... "Am I Safe?"

Your brain is constantly asking that question and it certainly applies to movement.

Physical training should be about improving one or more of the following core elements:

Stability

Mobility

Strength

Power

Conditioning

Endurance

Stamina

Agility

Quickness

Why? Because you owe it to yourself to honour the vehicle you inhabit, respecting yourself enough to appreciate that your body is the only one you have and it is your responsibility to make sure you move with purpose on a daily basis. Focusing on these elements allows you to experience more out of life by giving you the confidence in your own ability to tackle whatever comes your way.

The problem is, so many people get caught up in the latest exercise fad, usually in the hope of losing weight, without adjusting anything else in their lifestyle. Let's be clear, you cannot out train a bad diet. It requires way too much effort for little return. For example, beverages from coffee shops can range anywhere from 400-1000 calories. Liquid calories are quick to consume. To put it in context, to burn those calories off would take anywhere from 1-2 hours exercise. That's without considering the impact on your hormonal balance. Coffee and sugar will send you on a stimulant rollercoaster that over time has a definite impact on your health.

Anyway, let's get back to movement. I just want to make it clear, that moving more (with purpose) is only one aspect of optimising your health.

Fitness is really about optimising all the elements in the list just mentioned.

Fuelling your body with the right type of food optimises your health, reduces body fat and changes body composition.

| 8 |

Creating a Training Program

Just as I see health as a jigsaw, physical movement can be seen this way too. Creating a training program involves a number of elements that all 'fit' together. The picture isn't complete if any of the pieces are missing.

To be clear, 'weight training' is not a training program. It is a tool used as part a complete fitness program. Similarly, cardio is not a training program but another piece of a complete fitness program.

For many people, working out and training are the same. Whatever it takes to get the heart pumping and the blood flowing, whether that is going to the gym or going for a run.

But exercise and training programs are different things. It's how you approach the activity, not the activity itself.

What is exercise?

Exercise is something that enhances or maintains physical fitness as part of your overall health and wellness. Exercising moderately 30 minutes per day, 5 days a week is a good rule of thumb, the fundamental goal being to improve cardiovascular capacity (fitness), immune system function, brain health, sleep quality and mental wellbeing.

What is training?

Why is this different to exercise? Training is a systematic approach to a specific outcome, an intention to actively improve something in a physical way, just like you would train to increase flexibility through stretching or training your mind through meditative practice or throwing punches and kicks in martial arts. The point is to work towards improving something, to condition yourself to operate at a higher level.

Whether you should be exercising or training comes down to your specific goals. Exercising is choosing an activity that brings enjoyment and gets your heart pumping. However, if you want to improve strength, stamina, endurance, agility, quickness, and flexibility for a specific purpose then you need a training program.

These things just don't happen as a result of general exercise and movement but from a predictable response to routinely putting your body under increased demand over time. That requires a plan.

I see so many people who want 'training' results from 'exercising'. There has to be a plan, something that can be tracked can be measured and when it can be measured it can be tweaked and adjusted. Otherwise how would you know how to improve?

A complete program should include:

Movement preparation. A way of preparing the body to move with purpose to develop stability, mobility and range of motion safely.

Power and elasticity. Many people think this is just for athletes, however we lose these qualities the fastest with aging so it is important to include them in your training program.

Core. Direct and indirect movements to test and improve the strength of your midsection.

Strength. A big part of a training program but not the only part. Improving strength boosts your metabolic rate, movement control, immunity and increases bone density, functional strength and cardio-vascular health. It gives you a big bang for your buck.

Metabolic or Cardio. Most people benefit from some form of direct cardiovascular activity. It doesn't have to be traditional cardio such as running, but what you do still has to have a purpose. Whether that is general conditioning, general physical preparedness, endurance/stamina or agility and quickness, your body will benefit from it all.

This template helps you create a balanced approach to moving effectively with purpose. However, it is essential that you start from where your body is currently capable of safely.

| 9 |

Recovery

One thing that is important to remember. You get better by RECOV-ERING from training. Training is just the catalyst; it's a stressor that basically breaks down the body. We get weaker temporarily and then the body adapts and comes back stronger.

All the training sessions in the world don't mean a thing if you don't allow yourself sufficient time to recover. You have to allow the body to recover and adapt to the stimulus. The harder and longer the stimulus, the longer the recovery will be.

Here are a few things to remember to help you get the most of your exercise/training:

1. **Train smart with structured, progressive training programs.**

   This doesn't mean you don't train hard, but being aware that working harder or longer means your recovery period can take longer. Always be aware of the impact of adding more.

2. **Get the basics right**

   Have enough rest, sleep, hydration, protein and energy intake. It's important to get the foundations right. Even if your focus is fat loss, having an understanding of how to fuel your body and not to deprive it is vital.

3. **Look after your soft tissue**

   Flexibility, mobility, massage, foam rolling and Epsom / magnesium baths are all extremely useful tools that by and large get ignored. If you are continually breaking down muscle tissue when exercising, make sure you show it some love when rebuilding.

4. **Supplementation**

   One of the most common issues is that of deficiencies, but think of vitamins and mineral supplements as nutrients without calories. They fill in the gaps to make sure you have all the bases covered. Your body can only repair itself with the fuel you give it so make sure that is high quality most of the time.

5. **Low intensity activity**

   Rest and recovery are important, but that doesn't mean to say lying around is optimal for recovery. Some form of low intensity activity can help the recovery process. There is nothing wrong with planned rest days, however low intensity aerobic work, foam rolling or a mobility session can actually speed up recovery.

It's important to remember, you get better by recovering FROM training. Always consider less is often more. Any additional exercise is only better if it doesn't impede your recovery process.

Most people who have energy dips and feel burnt out are less likely to be suffering from over training and more likely to be from under recovery.

| 10 |

Bulletproof Your Body

The missing element that most people don't consider when increasing movement, is whether your body feels safe. It is constantly assessing whether how you move is safe or not.

If your body does not feel safe, in this case stable, it will do whatever it takes to create stability. As I have mentioned in a previous chapter, the body will tighten muscles and it will compress or lock joints, even if this leads to the production of pain. Your central nervous system does all it can to protect you, even if it results in pain.

Pain is your body's last course of action which comes after compensation after compensation does not work. Pain is a more immediate response to threat, something deemed by the brain to be unsafe and may cause harm so the brain makes it hurt because it doesn't want you to do it.

This is why I believe it is madness to embark on an exercise program without first having your movement assessed. This could be some form of movement screen such as the Functional Movement Screen (created by Gray Cook), or some other screening method. It is always prudent to see where you start from to optimise your movement. If there are any 'red flags' highlighted don't push through them. Seek advice from a good physical therapist first. It is better to be clear on your start point, so you can build a solid foundation from which to create safe movement patterns. This will minimise pain and niggles down the line.

Generic exercise routines without any regard to the individual can ultimately result in injury. The first rule in any exercise or training program should be to do no harm, so find a coach or trainer who has your best interests and safety in mind. That is only possible if you are assessed as an individual.

Too many times I have had conversations with people who have come to me in pain having been injured because of some crazy exercise routine from YouTube they have undertaken without any kind of assessment or movement preparation (warm up) before they started.

So what happens when you find yourself in pain?

There are many reasons, but developing dysfunctional movement patterns can create reduced movement and increased pain.

If you have had any trauma or injury (maybe you have sprained an ankle or broken your foot or fallen out of a tree when you were young) or if you have been physically injured, the motor control centre (MCC) in your brain will change your movement pattern to compensate for the injury to still allow you to move whilst keeping you mobile and safe from harm.

The MCC stores all the coordination patterns of the body. It is directed by the limbic system in your brain to create movement patterns (such as when a baby learns to stand and walk) and also to create substitute movement patterns when you are injured.

After healing, your motor control centre doesn't automatically go back to using the original movement patterns. If the perceived pain hasn't been rehabbed, the MCC continues to use the compensations it created. This is the most frequent cause of pain and weakness.

The MCC has to be reprogrammed to use the right muscles for the right movement patterns. This can be done by physical therapists who have the correct skills to find the root cause of the initial problems not just treat the symptoms. At a basic level, this means understanding manual muscle testing to see what muscles are overworking so they can be released (muscles can be tight and weak from overworking) and finding the corresponding underactive muscles and activating them. It's no use releasing muscles without knowing why they are overworking in the first place and activating them, otherwise the MCC goes back to the old dysfunctional patterns. It's amazing what the body can tell you if you have the awareness to listen.

I have worked with so many people who have suffered unnecessary pain for a long time. One client felt weak down the right side of her body for years, especially when exercising. Amazingly, she had stubbed her left big toe when she was 5 years old and her body had compensated for that injury by over using her right side to keep her away from the pain. Even though her toe had healed years before, the new dysfunctional movement pattern had 'stuck' and had remained there for 50 years!

Scars are another potential big problem and can completely change how you move. I worked with another client who had had knee reconstructions and was unaware that the scarring had switched off muscles and created dysfunctional patterns. He had not been correctly assessed for rehab so these compensations had gone unnoticed and led to further injuries. Eventually, by looking at the deeper issues and using the physical symptoms as a guide led to understanding why the body felt unsafe and helped create stability by finding the original cause. The client in question thought it was voodoo magic!

Just because you have knee pain for example, doesn't mean to say you have knee problems. 95% of knee pain is to do with your hips and / or ankle issues.

The knee for example, can bear the brunt of dysfunctional movement patterns in the joints above or below the knee. So when you see a physical therapist who just focuses on the site of pain beware, most if not all pain is referred pain from somewhere else in the body.

So be mindful of past injuries, pains and niggles and understand that your body doesn't automatically go back to correct movement patterns after injury. It has created more dominant movement patterns and compensations to help, allowing you move, but it is these same patterns that can hinder you long term and need to be addressed to allow pain free movement.

Prevention is always better than cure and resting rarely cuts it. Most pain is referred from problems elsewhere in the body, so it always makes sense to treat the underlying cause and not just the symptoms. Painkillers may simply mask the symptoms.

Remember muscles just do what they are told. There is a reason why they won't get any looser when you stretch them, or why if you go for a massage you just tighten straight back up.

If you treat the source of the pain, your symptoms are more likely to go away and stay away.

Corrective exercise

Once dysfunctional movement patterns are identified and are either re-programmed or cleared, any muscles imbalances or weakness can be addressed. Quite often, by diagnosing movement issues with a tool like the FMS, specific corrective exercises can be used to alleviate muscle imbalances, release overworking muscles, activate neurologically underworking 'switched off' muscles, allowing stability and mobility to return to the body. A stable body free of muscle and movement compensations will allow you to increase mobility and flexibility and build strength and fitness more effectively.

| 11 |

Stability and Mobility

Ever wonder how your body actually works? I have always been fascinated with how we move. That fascination started at school. I loved biology and finding out about how humans tick.

At 17, I was about to take my black belt grading in kick boxing. Part of the grading was to learn all the bones and muscles in the body and I was told to use a diagram so I could learn and list all their names.

I found a diagram, removed all the names and created 50 copies. Every day I wrote down what I could remember, looked at the original diagram and filled in the blanks. I figured if I did that every day for 50 days I would eventually remember. It worked too. It didn't even take 50 days. I was so determined to know every single one.

When I handed a blank drawing of the bones and muscles to my karate instructor, he told me the exam was to consist of random questions about human anatomy. I had not been expected to know all the names of the individual bones and muscles.

I asked for a pen and filled out every bone and muscle on my blank sheet, right in front of my amazed instructor. I guess I got some brownie points for being studious!

Suffice to say, I passed my grading and got my first black belt aged 17. I still remember that day. I was so proud of myself.

I believe it is always prudent and wise to understand your body and how it moves. Why this isn't taught at school I will never know. Why wouldn't you want to bring awareness to the amazing vehicle you inhabit and the importance of looking after it?

During all my years in martial arts, both training and coaching, I came to realise that I can improve the performance of myself and others by understanding more about physiology and anatomy and how it all works together.

I can only share what I found out, what worked and what makes sense to me. Understanding where someone's current movement level is and starting them from that point is crucial to minimise the risk of injury.

How do we define mobility?

Quite simply put, mobility is how far you can move a joint under your own body's control without any external influence; the ability to move freely

How do we define stability?

With mobility in mind, stability is how well you can control the mobility you have. If you have a lack of stability the brain will limit your mobility through a joint if it deems it unstable to prevent injury. If the body doesn't feel a movement is safe it won't allow you to move.

Joint by joint approach.

This approach was popularised by an American strength coach called Michael Boyle and a movement specialist called Gray Cook.

The idea is that each joint has a role or purpose, to either to stabilise or mobilise. The first major joint from the floor is your ankle. That joint has a lot of range of movement and is classed as a mobility joint. The next up is your knee, which is more of a stability joint having less range of motion than the ankle. After that is the hip, which again can move in many directions and is a mobility joint. This carries on up the kinetic chain. Your lower back or lumbar spine is all about stability, your thoracic spine (mid back) mobility, your scapular or shoulder blade is all about stability and your shoulder joint mobility. Notice the switch between mobility and stability.

However, if one of these joints or the area around a joint suffers trauma such as a sprain, strain or poor posture, the body moves to stabilise the joint to protect it and flips the function of that joint. The thing is, by doing so it can flip the function of each other joints in the chain. So if you injure your ankle, the body moves to change this mobile joint to a stable one. This has the knock on effect of changing the knee from a stability joint to a mobility joint and so on up the chain.

Over time, since the knee is not built for that kind of movement, it can result in knee pain. That is why it is important to assess not just the symptoms of pain, but why they could be there, what is the causation? It's not always the site of the pain that is the issue, most often it is referred from somewhere else.

The three most common global compensation patterns the body uses to create stability in a movement are holding your breath, clenching your jaw or the use of the calf muscles. Any one of these can be used in a dysfunctional movement pattern to help stabilise you. Have you ever noticed holding your breath or clenching your jaw when trying to perform an action such as opening a jar?

If you have joint pain then please seek professional help from a physical therapist who understands how to find the cause of the issue (see resources section in the book for more information).

What does this mean for you?

Your system is all about safety. That is its number one priority and movement is no exception. The body will only allow you full mobility in a movement if it feels stable doing so. So many people go about their life unaware that poor posture and poor movement coupled with any past injuries can restrict your movement and cause pain. Injury prevention and pain management are about getting the body to function normally and optimally. When working on the body to achieve full range of motion and mobility, control is essential for everyday movement.

| 12 |

Stretching vs Flexibility

Being a martial artist of over 30 years I have encountered many ways to stretch, some good, some not so much. I have seen some brutal stretching methods that have no place in any dojo, doing more harm than good. Without any real knowledge of how muscles work, it can be dangerous, simply because everyone is an individual with a history. Listen to your body and don't push through any unnecessary pain.

Yoga or Pilates are good ways to increase movement and flexibility or specific stretching classes with experienced instructors.

One thing I do know is, there is a time and a place for stretching.

When your body feels safe, when it feels stable, your body is more likely to allow you to stretch. I have seen martial artists who cannot reach down to their knees, never mind to touch their toes and yet can kick head height with ease. Why is that? Because bending forward was an unsafe movement. The body didn't feel stable and so tightened muscles to protect itself, however the movement of kicking head height felt safe.

Safety

Why does your brain take away movement? To keep you from moving. Simple right?

Why does it keep you from moving? Because it's not stable/safe.

To get mobility in joints, and flexibility in muscles you better back it up with stability. Getting mobility and flexibility isn't the hard part. Keeping it is.

3 states a muscle can be in.

1. Normal movement – The muscles can fully contract, lengthen and relax, meaning it's stretchable.
2. Muscles that don't switch off – Muscles are overactive, usually tight and weak from trying to stabilise a joint.
3. Muscles that don't switch on – Muscles are neurologically underactive.

3 ways to look at stretching.

1. Stretches can increase your range of motion. Your brain is allowing you to train at an increased range of motion. This is how it is supposed to work. Your brain needs to feel safe when increasing the range of motion of a muscle.
2. Try to stretch and nothing changes, the muscle feels tight with no give. Be aware that flexibility is granted, it's not trainable. If your brain perceives it needs tightness in a muscle to feel safe then it will not allow you to stretch the muscle. Forcing it can often lead to injury.
3. Some stretch, some give, but it makes things worse and your muscles end up tighter than before. More than likely taking away a compensation that is helping create stability around a joint. So

if you remove compensation problems, things could get worse until you add the compensation back or remove the issue.

That's when you have to and find out why the muscle is tight. Remember, muscles do what they are told so if there is no give or they tighten back up they are doing so in response to the brain telling them to do that, to protect something and feel safe. That's why it is so important to find a physical therapist who can explain how your body works, and how to safely stretch without injury. If the brain feels it's not safe for muscles to stretch then it will not allow it until the issue is resolved. Don't force it.

So many people assume tight muscles need stretching, but unless you correctly assess the opposite could be true. Muscles can be tight AND weak, meaning they are providing a compensation, holding on to keep things moving. This is most often what leads to injury.

Many people suffer from something called anterior pelvic tilt. This is when your pelvis tilts forward and can lead to symptoms such as lower back pain or tight hamstrings (the muscles at the back of your thighs). This is most common in sedentary people, who sit down most of the day and do little exercise or movement.

Remember, your body wants to be efficient at what it does the most, so if that is sitting, it will change the angle of your pelvis, shorten your hip flexors (the muscles in front of your hips that help raise the knee) and it will switch off your glutes (butt muscles) which all lead to that pelvic tilt.

So if you have anterior pelvic tilt and have tight hamstrings, stretching your hamstrings without having been assessed makes no sense. You may get temporary relief, but you have given the pelvis more chance to tilt forward and made the problem worse. Learning why the tilt exists and by knowing what muscles are underworking and what muscles are overworking, you are able to perform exercises to rectify the problem to allow you to stretch safely.

It's all about finding out why muscles are tight. That's when you must seek professional help.

A red flag for me is when a therapist doesn't investigate. They focus on the site of the pain without investigating what may be causing the pain and giving exercises that could actually make the problem worse.

With that in mind here are some things to consider when starting a stretching routine

1. **There is a difference between flexibility and stretching.**
   Flexibility is the ability for soft tissue including muscles, tendons and ligaments to lengthen correctly and safely. Stretching is a form of exercise that can lead to increased flexibility.

2. **Flexibility is subjective.**
   Depending on an individual's injury history and posture, muscles could be stiff or tight. It's easy to think that a tight muscle needs stretching. Make sure the body isn't keeping it tight for a reason.

3. **Static stretching**
   Performed without movement usually in a relaxed manner. Unless you are working to increase flexibility in sports such as martial arts, static stretching should be performed after exercise as part of a cool down as warm muscles are less likely to tear. Stretching statically before exercising can weaken the muscle and lead to injury.

4. **Dynamic stretching**
   Performed with movement such as swinging or bouncing to extend the range of motion and flexibility. This is more suited to warm ups and is more effective in preparing your body to move.

5. **Don't over stretch**
   Holding a stretch to improve your flexibility, assuming your

muscles are functional with normal movement is fine. However don't hold a stretch to a point of pain, just to a point of mild discomfort.

6. **Ask a professional**

Find a qualified professional who can advise the correct type of stretching for you. Everyone is unique with stability, mobility and flexibility and different injury histories. A combination of dynamic, static movements are meant to improve your movement, not hinder it.

Always make sure you know your body's capabilities before you start a stretching program. Check in with a physical therapist who understand movement. See resources section for more details of recommended physical therapies.

| 13 |

The Health Pyramid

I believe there are three main areas we get to focus on in order to formulate the foundation of optimal health...

Your gut, your blood sugar balance and how you manage stress.

Each one is interlinked and if any one of them is out of balance, if will affect the others.

Let's explore each one in turn to see how the work synergistically and how they affect us when they don't.

| 14 |

Looking After Your Gut

We are what we ingest and absorb. Everything we consume becomes us. It's so easy to eat whatever your taste buds fancy, but every action has a consequence and if you are not honouring yourself with good food (at least most of the time) then the bill becomes due.

I see gut health as a vital part of improving our overall health. Of the three main areas in the pyramid where we optimise health, the gut is the most important as it can manipulate the other systems, namely blood sugar management and adrenal function or stress management. They all go hand in hand.

So let's take a quick look to show you why it is so important.

- Did you know the Gut is over 22 feet long and runs from your mouth to your anus?
- It has its own nervous system known as the Enteric Nervous System, which actually has MORE nerve cells than your spinal column. This is why the gut is referred to as our second brain.
- It houses 75% of your total immune system in or around it.
- Over 400 different species of bacteria (that we know of) are in the gut and balance is critical for your health.

- We have about 5-10lb of bacteria in the gut (gut flora)
- There are more bacteria in the gut than cells in the body.
- The gut actually is home to more neurotransmitters like serotonin and dopamine than the brain.

The gut is the barrier to the outside world, our first line of defence. The digestive system is actually external to the body. If our gut health is poor we increase the likelihood of picking up things like autoimmune diseases and viruses so it is vital to keep it healthy. Do not underestimate how important that is!

Bear in mind that 70% of autoimmune diseases are environmental, which means it's something we can take control of, for example lifestyle and emotional issues. It is important to really take responsibility for how you are living your life, not just the food that you eat. Question what you are really in control of and whether you are allowing other influences to affect how you think and feel.

It is important for you to be aware of and understand any potential problems and identify solutions to help you thrive.

Gut Health and Gut Flora

Most people are not aware that it is the bacteria, or more importantly the balance of good and bad bacteria in our gut that protects us from pathogens and other foreign bodies. This is what is known as gut flora. The key to gut health is maintaining the balance between good and bad.

Gut flora help maintain the integrity of the gut lining by secreting an antibody (IgA) which forms a protective layer to block harmful bacteria. This antibody plays a critical role in immunity and preventing infection.

Cells of the immune system are also prominent in the gut. They secrete chemical messengers known as cytokines that coordinate the inflammatory response in the body.

The gut flora can also assist in dealing with potential infections and also helps prevent allergies by balancing the histamine response and down-regulating inflammation.

Inside the gut's mucus layers, thousands of hormone cells are produced that help aid digestion and metabolism. The trillions of microbes also play a vital role in nutrition because they synthesize vitamins such as thiamine, folic acid, pyridoxine, and vitamin K, as well as producing digestive enzymes that facilitate the absorption of calcium, magnesium, and iron.

Unfortunately, time, lifestyle, and environmental factors will ultimately degrade this complex system, unless you take steps to prevent it.

Gut Health Imbalances

What we eat plays an enormous role in maintaining the integrity of the gut and bacterial imbalance appears to be heavily influenced by diet.

Sugar, wheat gluten, dairy, additives and preservatives, pesticides, herbicides, hormones, and antibiotics all have an impact on the balance of good and bad bacteria.

Non-dietary influences include prescription and over-the-counter medications, such as anti-inflammatories (NSAIDS), stress (physical, psychological, or physiological), radiation, immune deficiencies, and aging.

As harmful bacteria levels rise, the intestines become more permeable, making them less likely to keep harmful pollutants out or aid in the absorption of nutrients.

Bacteria, toxins, and undigested proteins and fats can leak into the bloodstream and trigger an autoimmune reaction, which increases the levels of histamine, cortisol (stress hormone), and cytokines (inflammatory markers). This situation is often referred to as "leaky gut syndrome."

Although not a medical term, leaky gut syndrome is a growing problem that is not being properly addressed. Symptoms are often treated, without addressing the actual root cause.

Symptoms of leaky gut syndrome include

- Gastrointestinal complaints such as bloating, gas, reflux, constipation or diarrhoea
- Frequent illnesses
- Allergies
- Chronic sinusitis
- Slow metabolism
- Skin conditions such as eczema or psoriasis
- Joint pain
- Headaches
- Anxiety, and/or depression

When the health of the gut continues to decline, food sensitivities and autoimmune disorders can develop, causing all manner of issues and diseases as the body becomes more and more compromised and defenceless.

The Gut Brain Connection

To have a fully functioning and well-nourished brain, you have to have a fully nourished digestive system. Your gut has to be in great shape to withstand the rigours of modern life. Your brain is completely dependent on what you digest so if you cannot digest the nutrients your brain needs it will lead to poor brain function and inflammation.

We actually have two nervous systems...

Brain - Autonomic nervous system

Gut - Enteric nervous system

In early foetal development, the gut and brain originate from the same tissue before dividing, with one developing into the autonomic nervous system (brain) and the other developing into the enteric nervous system (digestive system). They remain connected by the vagus nerve from the brain stem to the stomach. They even share the same amount of neuro transmitters and hormones, each having around 100 million nerve cells. The digestive system could even run on its own if it had a blood supply!

If your gut isn't happy, there is more than a good chance that your brain isn't happy. If your gut health is poor due to excess alcohol, coffee, sugar or pain killers or through frequent infections or antibiotics, your gut health will be compromised and you will most likely react to the food you eat, which will have an effect on your brain health.

Because the two systems are linked so closely, conditions such as a leaky gut can lead to brain issues, which can dramatically affect your mood, attention and behaviour. The most common and most undiagnosed immune and toxic reactions are caused by wheat gluten and dairy products.

The inflammation and toxic effects of gluten and casein, from wheat and dairy, are so powerful in affecting brain function that it can lead to anything from brain fog to depression.

The link between the gut and the brain is clear. What you eat has a direct effect on your brain, which means it can affect your mood and behaviour. A healthy gut will produce up to 90% of your body's serotonin, the happy neuro transmitter. With poor gut health, your body simply doesn't get enough. Your behaviour is influenced by what you eat and digest!

Food Transition

Think for a minute about the journey of the food we consume through the digestive system. Let's be honest, it is a marvellous process when you think about it.

This is the journey:

Chewing our food – Digestion starts in the mouth and prepares the stomach for what is about to come. That is why it is important to chew your food thoroughly. Salivary amylase from saliva starts digesting any simple carbohydrates contained in the food you are chewing.

Stomach – The primary function of the stomach is to churn and sanitise food. There are four muscles in the stomach designed to help with the breakdown primarily of proteins using an enzyme called pepsin.

Small intestine – There are three parts; the top part, liver and gallbladder produce bile at this point that helps breakdown and emulsifying of any fats that have been consumed. They are also involved in the breaking down of protein and carbs to their smallest possible parts to make absorption easier.

Large intestine – Deals mostly with the waste to be excreted. At this point the body absorbs the excess water and electrolytes from the matter before we pass it out.

Food transition times...

To give you an idea, the time it takes for food to move through your digestive system is around 12-16 hours. If digestion falls out of those times then there can be potential issues. What you ingest stays in the stomach for around 1-3 hours depending on the combination of food. After that it is the movement from the small to large intestines.

Why is this important to know?

Too short, i.e. less than 12 hours can point to deficiencies. Too long, i.e. greater than 16 hours points to digestive issues. If the time gets past 24 hours, that can lead to the body trying to reuptake and absorb what is in our intestines that can lead to other issues.

Potential Problems

There are three primary issues that affect gut health, deficiencies, infections and inflammation. Any of these three can affect upset the balance of the gut and if it affects your gut, it will have an impact on your brain.

Deficiencies

There are a few things to consider; Low HCL (stomach acid) is a common issue for many with stress being a major factor. Stress puts us in our sympathetic nervous system (Fight or flight response). Blood moves away from stomach to limbs ready to fight or run.

When stress goes up, HCL goes down leading to less sterilisation of food, less breakdown of food such as proteins, which can lead to autoimmune responses. Also when HCL is low there is an increased chance of pathogens and viruses getting past this sterilisation barrier.

Medications can cause low stomach acid too, things like antacids can potentially lower HCL when it wasn't high in the first place.

We can bring ourselves back into the para sympathetic nervous system also known as the rest and digest nervous system by utilising deep breathing, see the 'I Can't Get No Sleep' chapter for more details.

It is so important to have balanced gut flora. With the pill popping culture and poor health that is so prevalent these days, it's common to look for the quick fix or magic pill. There isn't one, so stop looking. Give your body what it needs and optimise your lifestyle.

Infections

Infections are more common than you think and not easy to detect by conventional (read modern medical) means. They can affect the small intestines with things such as SIBO (small intestine bacterial overgrowth) and large intestines too. Over time they can become chronic and cause systemic inflammation, which can lead to all kinds of disease.

Types of infection

There are different types of infections including bacterial, yeast, fungal and parasitic.

Infections can mimic diseases, for example parasitic infections can mimic autoimmune disease symptoms. These can affect the lining of the large intestines. The surface of the large intestine is covered by finger like projections called villi, which in turn have micro villi then brush boarders. Celiac disease for example flattens the villi which leads to poor absorption and the possibility of increased pain. An example of symptoms include increased mucus, which stops the breakdown of food causing fermentation, leading to gas, bloating, pain and distention.

Parasitic infections are also problematic as they take from the host and manipulate the host for their own gain. Parasites live in different stages and can be active and inactive in their growth cycle which makes them hard to detect and a lot of tests miss them. Conducting tests over a number of days is key as parasites can remain in the body for a long time.

Something to consider if you have had long term undiagnosed health issues. If you have been to a third world country and been ill and had sickness and diarrhoea, there is a high likelihood of you having picked up a parasite.

Don't put up with not feeling right, regardless of what medics say. You know if you are not yourself. It just means you need a different tool for the job to diagnose the problem.

Inflammation

You can find out more about this in the 'Inflammation' chapter. Suffice to say there are 3 things to consider that can lead to inflammation; allergies, intolerances and sensitivities.

These can be caused by things like medication, alcohol, drugs, poor food choices, emotional stress, which can all affect gut health and creates an immune system response leading to inflammation. Reducing long term, chronic inflammation is key to reducing symptoms.

It is important to reduce inflammation as much as possible to allow your gut health to thrive.

The simplest way to find out whether you are reacting to the food you are eating is to perform an elimination diet; removing the most common allergenic foods for a number of days before reintroducing them one at a time to see how your body reacts.

Putting Good Gut Health into Practice

It is important to look after your gut. By removing toxins and toxic foods and including nourishing foods and supplements, you not only steer yourself away from diseases, bugs and disorders brought about by food allergies, sensitivities and intolerances, but you are also able to absorb more nutrients for your body and brain.

To make sure you are getting all your body needs for gut health it is important that you eat whole foods such as fresh vegetables and some fruits, lean meats, eggs and fish or protein alternatives in place of meat. Reduce or remove the toxic foods such as wheat and dairy, sugar, alcohol and caffeine. Also consider good quality nutritional supplements that help with gut health to make sure you remain symptom free.

Remove stress by practising mindful eating. It's important to create a calm and relaxed environment and create a positive experience at meal times by removing stress before eating.

Chew Your Food

Your digestion of food actually starts in your mouth. You produce up to 32 ounces of saliva each day. Chewing your food will help your body absorb vital nutrients more thoroughly and rapidly due to enzymes secreted in your saliva.

Eat slowly and chew your food at least 25 times per mouthful. Make sure it is a liquid pulp before swallowing. It takes 20 mins or so for the brain to register that you have eaten. This is why you should never eat when you are starving hungry as you will eat far more than you need. Taking your time and chewing slower lets your stomach signal your brain to say, right I am full, so you stop taking in excess calories.

Your tongue recognises various flavours of each food and will send messages to the brain, which then tells your stomach to produce the corresponding digestive juices needed to break down that food.

So really our digestive system is about digestion, absorption and excretion. Mindful of eating, nourish your body with good food and make eating an experience.

| 15 |

Blood Sugar Rollercoaster

It may sound boring but understanding how important maintaining a good blood sugar balance is to your health will definitely have some light bulbs going off in your life. You may just connect some dots...

Blood glucose (sugar) management is another part of the health pyramid. So many people ride the daily blood sugar roller coaster through poor food choices and wonder why they feel so tired and irritable, not to mention struggling to lose weight, have any energy or have any quality sleep. Even if weight loss isn't a concern (and you would be in the minority) blood sugar regulation is hugely important.

Insulin is your storage hormone responsible for maintaining blood sugar balance in your blood and very important for getting energy to your cells. Its primary role is to keep blood glucose levels balanced. If your blood sugar is frequently too high or too low too often it will cause you all manner of health issues.

Let's not mix words here, in the most extreme circumstances it can be fatal. Blindness, seizures, brain damage and death are real if you neglect this long term. These are just some of the symptoms from diabetes. It's very important to understand what the role of insulin has for us.

What is Insulin?

Insulin is a peptide, it's a protein based hormone, and it's produced by an organ in the body called the pancreas. Insulin is released by the body when there's too much blood glucose in the bloodstream. Insulin is released to shuttle the excess glucose into the cells for energy within the skeletal muscle or to store later as fat. On the other hand, if blood sugar is too low, the pancreas releases glucagon, a hormone which brings the level of blood glucose levels up.

The body works hard to keep blood glucose in a tightly regulated healthy range so we always have fuel for our cells to use.

The problem we have is that the western diet has become very unhealthy. The sheer amount of refined sugars and processed foods that are consumed will cause blood sugar spikes and crashes. When we have a sugar crash, all kinds of feelings are displayed such as cravings and fatigue.

Because this diet is poor and devoid of nutrients, it can and often does cause a lot of stress and inflammation in the body. So we've got to be able to make sure that the body can regulate it effectively and there lies the problem. Sometimes it struggles to do that because of what we ingest. The adrenal glands fire cortisol to raise blood sugar when the body is under some form of stress, whether it needs the energy or not.

Because the brain runs on glucose as its main fuel source, if blood glucose dips and stays too low for too long and insulin can't deal with it then there is a danger of brain damage, seizures, even death.

Conversely, if you get the glucose levels too high then it becomes toxic and can lead to blindness and loss of limbs. This is commonly known as diabetes. It's something that so many people just don't even think about, mindless eating without any concern of the consequence of their actions over time. There is no concern whether it should be consumed, taking the view that if a supermarket sells it, it must be okay.

You get to take back control responsibility for the vehicle you inhabit. Good blood glucose management is important because it is a precursor to so many processes in the body. It provides the fuel to create energy in your cells. We can store glucose and glycogen in small amounts in the liver, some in the muscles and some in the blood so we've got energy for moving. After that it has to be regulated.

These days there is an epidemic level of high unregulated blood glucose levels in the blood for so many people.

That's why glucometers can be so invaluable in measuring blood glucose levels at various points in the day to see the reaction to what you are eating, where your energy is and your insulin response.

If you understand your own body, then you can improve your health and make it much better. Bringing awareness to what you are eating, how your body responds to what you eat, where your energy is at and how you are feeling are great indicators what to do next.

So if we think about how our metabolism works, eaten carbohydrates go into stomach and get digested, and then go into the small intestines to be broken down into their smallest possible form and absorbed through the intestine via the liver into the bloodstream. This stimulates the pancreas to release insulin when we eat excess carbohydrates. If blood glucose goes up then it's the role of insulin to bring it back down. Insulin keeps blood glucose levels into a range that's healthy and that is tightly controlled by the body.

Insulin can inhibit the release of glucose into the bloodstream if you don't require it. It acts on muscle tissue to help shuttle glucose into the cells to create ATP (our instant energy source). Insulin can help with increased fat storage, which is not something that you really want but if you've got high levels of insulin running because you're eating excess calories all the time, insulin can then provide the conversion to triglycerides (also known as fat) shuttling it to the fat cells to be used for energy later.

This is why if you eat too many excess calories from carbohydrates and your body doesn't need the fuel, then the body will store it.

If we're eating carbs all the time, why would your body then metabolise fat for energy? It's not going to expend energy metabolising fat from cells when there's energy in abundance already, so we've got to really think about what we're eating and the fact that we don't need energy dense carbohydrates such as potatoes, pasta or rice with every meal like so many people often do.

The western diet is loaded with sugar and highly processed food, which wreaks havoc on your body's blood sugar balance and that doesn't help us with shedding excess fat from our fat cells.

It also acts on the hormones leptin and ghrelin. Leptin is our fuel gauge to tell us when we are full and ghrelin signals when we are hungry. If we have dysregulated levels of insulin, then we can have dysregulated levels of leptin and ghrelin too. Everything impacts everything. Mixed signals can cause us to eat more than we need.

When we eat carbohydrates, they get broken down and digested and then absorbed by the bloodstream as glucose. Insulin shuttles glucose to the cell as fuel for our mitochondria, which are the energy batteries of every cell in the body enabling us to live.

Insulin is protein based, which makes it a problem for insulin to get the glucose into the cell directly. It needs help from fat based hormones, vitamins and minerals to pass through the cell membrane. Once in the cell, the cell receptors decide whether to use the glucose for energy or store it as fat.

Think of these receptors as doormen on a nightclub door, you ain't coming in if your name ain't down LOL. It is the receptors that come to the door and let glucose in. If we have too much insulin from elevated glucose levels for too long, the receptors downregulate, known as insulin resistance and that reduces the ability to take glucose into the cell. The longer this happens the more likely you will end up with type 2 diabetes.

You get to take responsibility for your health and manage your insulin levels by looking at your diet. The foods you consume have a direct bearing on your blood glucose management. Your body ultimately has control of that, but if your diet involves refined sugars, processed foods and energy drinks for example, you are not doing yourself any favours long term.

This impacts how you feel; high insulin levels affect your mood, hormone balance and your motivation to do things. If your blood sugar is all over the place from continually ingesting carbohydrates, your blood sugars will be on a roller coaster.

Sorting out your diet is one of the simplest things to do to stabilise and regulate blood sugar. Sticking to mostly protein and fat based meals with lots of colourful veggies will make a big difference.

Long term, high blood sugar levels raise inflammation as well. Cortisol is released with any kind of inflammation response because it's a stressor, a threat to the body. Anything that's a threat or unsafe to the body insulin gets released. The role of cortisol is to raise blood sugar levels as part of the fight or flight response, which is ok short term, but long term it becomes an issue.

This is why mindful eating and creating time to appreciate nourishing respect your body is important.

If we have unregulated high levels of insulin from poor diets, from high emotional and physical stress and not sleeping well that impacts blood sugar levels that has been proven to increase susceptibility to cancer, and cardiovascular disease.

The easiest way to measure blood sugar is with a glucometer, which measures the amount of glucose in your blood. You can measure your blood glucose levels on waking, before meal and after meal to get a good idea of how well your body is managing blood sugar.

Whether you're hypoglycaemic, which is low blood sugar or hyperglycaemic, high blood sugar, we're all susceptible to one or the other. There's no hard and fast rules as to which one it will be. It just depends on so many factors such as your sleep, stress environment, what we're eating etc. Regular checks are important.

Hypoglycaemia (Low Blood Sugar)

The usual signs for hypoglycaemia are feeling sluggish but perking up and feeling better after eating a meal. Eating meals closer together will help.

Also check what kind of carbohydrates you've had and have protein with every meal to create a longer sustainable, gentler sort of rise and fall of blood sugar. Exercise will definitely affect you as well. So it depends on the type of exercise.

Hyperglycaemia (High Blood Sugar)

Conversely, hyperglycaemia is high blood sugar. When you eat carbohydrates you suffer from fatigue and just want to go to sleep. This is a sign of insulin resistance because your body's not been able to clear out excess blood glucose because it's had too much for a long time. In this situation you would look at removing carbohydrates from the body by exercising to burn up the fuel and eating a lower carb diet.

So let's just recap.

Blood sugar and insulin are incredibly important and go hand in hand. We can easily eat too much too often, which causes insulin resistance, which in turn causes all manner of problems. Blood sugar and insulin can help or inhibit how we feel depending on how many carbohydrates we eat and whether we continue to do so in excess.

Low levels of blood sugar are very dangerous and can cause brain damage and seizures. Your brain needs glucose to function. Too high levels cause serious conditions such as type two diabetes, joint issues, blindness or loss of limbs. Your blood sugar has to be kept in a tight range without insulin having to pull it up or down because of overconsumption.

The more we allow it to go up and down, creating rapid rises and big crashes through our diet and what we ingest, the more the likelihood of insulin resistance will increase. So you really have to get a handle on this.

If insulin is in the appropriate range, inflammation in your body will lower, it will regulate itself and your body will start functioning better. Unfortunately poor diets are common these days in the western world. There is so much pressure on our body from stress, the foods we eat, the environmental exposures we experience such as car fumes, pesticides and herbicides and a lack of quality sleep.

It's rare that our body can handle everything. Sometimes we need to intervene. Optimising our diet, reducing stress and regulating blood glucose gives you back control of your body to improve your health. Doing so creates better insulin sensitivity, better mood, better body composition, less chance of cardiovascular disease, cancer or other degenerative diseases.

A lot of what we're eating in general in the western world is quite toxic, and change is our responsibility. You get to take back control of your blood sugar and respect the vehicle you inhabit.

| 16 |

The Stress Response

The third and final part of the health pyramid.

We all know how stress feels right?

Long term chronic stress can be caused by a number of factors; the adrenal glands, the stress hormone cortisol and the regulated hormones all play their part.

Modern life moves way too fast and our bodies just aren't keeping up. Financial, relationship, work, nutritional, environmental, emotional and digestive stress are just some of the things that are having a major impact on our health.

Left out of control, chronic stress will wreak havoc on our immune, nervous, hormonal, emotional and musculoskeletal systems. Bad stressors can throw the body out of balance and can lead to internal overload and the breakdown of coping mechanisms. This in turn leads to diseases and disorders. Make no mistake chronic stress is hugely detrimental to your health and can kill if it's ignored.

The body is incredibly complex. Whilst we get on day by day living our lives, we are oblivious to the constant struggle of our bodies to keep things in balance.

The thing is, our bodies are simply not set up for this fast pace world we find ourselves in. We are in danger of being burnt out by the stressful living we all seem to endure day in day out.

We evolved in nature and this is how our body still tries to act out. We are too busy living in memories of the past or living in anticipation of the future to take time to slow down and live for the present.

Our Nervous System

The nervous system plays an important role in processing and evaluating stress in the body. Our nervous system is made up of 2 parts:

Peripheral – this system controls conscious movement

Autonomic – this system controls the actions in the body that are not from conscious thought such as breathing, digestion, sweating and releasing hormones.

The autonomic nervous system is split into 2 sub-systems:

Sympathetic Nervous System

The sympathetic nervous system (SNS) when activated triggers our fight or flight response. When threatened our natural instinct is to fight to protect ourselves or to run for our lives.

This brings about the release of the stress hormone cortisol to elevate heart rate, mobilise energy and increase blood pressure. It takes blood away from your internal organs to your skin and muscles, increases sweating and stops digestion.

Our primal survival instinct is the fight or flight response. When we are put under threat or stress our brains think our lives are in danger and our survival response kicks in. It simply cannot distinguish between a sabre toothed tiger chasing us thousands of years ago or the threat of a company deadline looming or presenting in front of hundreds of people. The response is identical.

Parasympathetic Nervous System

The parasympathetic nervous system (PNS) is where the body resides when you are in balance or in homeostasis. Also known as the rest and digest cycle, it supports the digestive and repair processes to replenish and rebuild your body.

In times of stress however, your PNS is constantly shut down, which is the common cause of a multitude of chronic fatigue states as well as emotional imbalances and distress. The PNS is where we should spend most of our time but frequently don't.

The Good and the Bad

We have what can be labelled good and bad stress, in reality these are labels based on perception. But what does that mean?

A 'good' type of stress is an acute short term stress, such as exercise, where training for shorter periods can be a good stress on the body.

But there's also long term 'bad' stress to consider.

Long term chronic stress can cause lots of problems in the body and can affect so many different systems, some of which you might even be struggling with right now.

It is responsible for two different types of stress that we can have.

So let's break it down into two stages:

Sympathetic Nervous System Response

The first stage is a sympathetic nervous response or the fight or flight response. When the limbic system is responding to something, maybe it's a car crash, or you see some form of danger or feel unsafe, you have this instantaneous fight of flight response.

When we are in this state we start getting an increase in blood pressure; we start to get an increase in blood sugars because we mobilise stored glycogen energy from the liver; our digestive function shuts down as blood is shuttled away from the stomach towards the extremities of your limbs. It makes you a machine for increased energy and increased action to keep you safe. Your eyes dilate so that you can actually have a wider field of vision. You even flatten the lens on your eye so you can actually see better and further.

This instantaneous response is really a life-saving mechanism for you and for acute short term stress is something that you absolutely need to happen.

Of course, nowadays in the western world, the same reactions are triggered for things like losing our job, having an argument or paying bills, when our ancestors were may have been running away from sabre toothed tigers.

Hormonal response

The second part of this response, the hormonal response is slower, but will be longer lasting. This response begins in the hypothalamus in the brain. The hypothalamus is responsible for many bodily functions including your emotions. As part of the stress response, it uses feedback from the nervous system and hormones to speak to the pituitary gland, which will then send a signal the adrenal glands to produce the stress hormone cortisol, and something called aldosterone.

The job of cortisol primarily is to raise blood sugars. It acts on the liver to mobilise glycogen, turning it into glucose to use for energy.

It gives you that boost so you can run away or fight or whatever you need to do to survive.

The job of aldosterone really is to act upon the kidneys to help reabsorb salt to help raise blood pressure and help us circulate things around the body.

So now we've introduced cortisol, let's look at why high cortisol and low cortisol can impact your health.

High Cortisol

If we have elevated levels of cortisol, there are a few things that we really need to pay attention to.

Because cortisol acts to raise your blood sugars, you will have an increased level of appetite and more likely to crave sugary, refined foods.

Remember, the primary role of cortisol is to help mobilise energy for fuel.

Having elevated levels of cortisol long term will create lower levels of muscle mass. Why is that an issue? Having lower levels of muscle mass can create a lower level of metabolism, therefore, things like fat loss would become more challenging.

Cortisol is also linked to lowering your level of a particular immune cell (IgA) that lines the gut. The higher level of cortisol, the lower level of the immune cell as cortisol acts a suppressant. The issue of having higher levels of cortisol and lower levels of the immune cell is that you open yourself up for infections. This immune cell is the first line of defence for your body. If cortisol is high we will reduce our level of protection and open ourselves up to certain pathogens or issues that we can have that come from foods or contaminated water for example.

Cortisol has always been known to act upon the pituitary. Remember the hypothalamus sends signals to the pituitary and the pituitary gland sends lots of hormones to glands and organs in the body in order to tell them to do what they need to do.

One of those glands is the thyroid.

Essentially, a signal from the hypothalamus tells the pituitary to send thyroid stimulating hormone (TSH) to the thyroid for in order to release thyroid hormones T4 and T3.

The production and release of thyroid hormone in the thyroid gland is regulated by a feedback loop, creating a dynamic balance, continually controlling the levels of thyroid hormones you need.

Every cell in the body has receptors for thyroid hormone. These hormones impact virtually every system in the body and are responsible for most basic aspects of bodily functions.

Importantly, thyroid hormones increase the metabolic rate of almost every tissue in the body. If you can imagine the thyroid gland as a furnace and the pituitary gland as the thermostat and thyroid hormones are like heat. When the heat gets back to the thermostat it switches off, until the temperature drops and so the thyroid once more is fired up once more sending thyroid hormones round the body.

Assuming the endocrine system is healthy and functional, this goes off without a hitch.

However, TSH can be blocked if you have high levels of cortisol. You can be showing all the symptoms of low thyroid function, or thyroid issues and it might actually be nothing to do with your thyroid. It might actually be to do with stress and elevated levels of cortisol that are blocking this pathway and therefore you display symptoms such as feeling sluggish or being unable to lose weight.

Cortisol can also downregulate the function of your thyroid gland by blocking the conversion of T4 to T3. T4 is the inactive form of your thyroid hormone that regulates your metabolism and has to be converted to activate your T3 for the body to use it. The problem when you are stressed is that cortisol blocks that conversion from T4 to T3, therefore your metabolism will be slower. That means that you could struggle with a lack of energy and fat loss.

High cortisol has been shown to affect your hippocampus which is responsible for converting short to long term memory. So think of all these neurodegenerative issues and diseases that we have nowadays. It's absolutely possible the high elevated levels of cortisol over a very long period of time are massively impacting what is happening in people's long term brain health.

People having high cortisol can display as skin issues, there may be visceral fat issues there might be insulin issues might be even memory issues too.

Low Cortisol

Now let's go to low cortisol.

Low cortisol something that is linked to things like depression, and pain and nausea, seasonal affective disorder, or SAD and Fibromyalgia or chronic fatigue. For example, people who take forever to recover from training sessions or just get wiped out via movement or activity and the body is very slow to regenerate, could be displaying signs of low cortisol.

Blood sugar issues are a big thing with low cortisol. Remember, one of the main actions of cortisol is to raise blood sugar. If you don't have enough cortisol, then blood sugar can start going below the ideal ranges. This is very dangerous to the brain as glucose is the brains primary fuel source. If you have lower levels, you can start getting very irritable and dizzy. So the ability to lose weight, to regulate your mood and deal with things like inflammation which is very tightly regulated into the immune system is very challenging.

It's common to blame 'adrenal fatigue', a term used when cortisol is low. But starting with the adrenals isn't the first place to look. The adrenals are told what to do and adrenal function can be affected by your immune system, gut health and inflammation to name a few. Any one of these will trigger the adrenals which will raise cortisol. But if we look at the causes, the symptoms will go away.

How would you know if you have low cortisol?

If after having laid down for 10 or 15 minutes, you get up and you feel lightheaded and dizzy you may have low cortisol because your blood pressure is regulated by cortisol and rebalancing should happen pretty effortlessly with no issues.

Before you jump to any conclusions it's important to review your lifestyle. Asking yourself what could actually be causing that response?

Are you stressed? Is it just emotional, mental? Is it physiological? Do you have some infections in your body? How is your sleep, is your sleep/wake cycle optimal? Do you have some inflammation in your body that isn't being dealt with?

Always start with why.

Steps to Reduce and Manage Stress

Identify the primary stressor. Focus on reducing stress is the area it is affecting you the most. The general priority from our brains in a stressful state is feeling safe, eating and procreation. Identifying and alleviating the chief stressor usually dramatically reduces other stressors.

Sleep – Aim to get at least 8 hours of quality sleep per night. Sleep is MASSIVELY underrated. Lack of good sleep can lead to excessive daytime tiredness and lethargy, morning headaches, poor memory, anxiety and depression. Remember Cortisol follows a similar sleep pattern. If you continually disrupt it you will become more stressed. Even better get into bed by 10:30pm.

Eat to nourish your body – Poor food choices place a huge stress on our digestive system. Internal stressors will only magnify external stressors. Removing fatty, sugary and processed foods and eating healthy foods such as fresh meats, vegetables (especially green leafy veg), fruits (mostly berries), nuts and seeds provides your body with all the nutrients it requires to maintain good health.

Drink more water – All of our organs, especially our brains, need water to function properly. If you're dehydrated, your body won't function optimally and that can lead to stress. Studies have shown that being just half a litre dehydrated can increase your stress levels.

Avoid Caffeine – Caffeine is a stimulant that increases adrenaline in the body, the very hormone you are looking to reduce. It adds to your symptoms and burns out your adrenals even faster when coupled with the stress you are already under. Instead go for a glass of water or herbal tea. One of the best teas to have is Tulsi tea, well known for its stress-lowering effects.

Exercise – Even 10 - 15 minutes of exercise will help bring your stress levels down. A High Intensity Interval workout would be best if other areas of stress were ok. However even going for a short walk, doing some stretching or breathing exercises will help. Exercise also produces endorphins, which are chemicals in the brain that creates a feel good feeling.

Diaphragmatic Breathing – Most people breath dysfunctionally, which adds to their stress. Stress activates your sympathetic nervous system. The goal of diaphragmatic breathing is to focus your awareness on your breath, making it slower and deeper. When you breathe in deeply through your nose, your lungs fully expand and your belly rises. This helps your heart rate slow down, allowing you to feel more peaceful. Deep breathing exercises can help activate your parasympathetic nervous system, which controls the relaxation response.

Turn off your mobile phone – Give yourself a break from your mobile phone. Most people have smart phones which can mean one-quarter of the working day is lost to interruptions from e-mails, phone calls and text messages, adding to stress. A failure to switch off from work is driving up stress levels. Put it on silent and check it 1-2 times a day.

Take Magnesium – Magnesium helps you to sleep restfully throughout the night and de-stress. Magnesium has a calming effect on the nervous system, meaning that if you are deficient your heart rate and sympathetic nervous system will be sent into overdrive. Additionally, lack of magnesium has shown to cause agitated sleep and frequent awakenings. Magnesium also makes your brain work better and improves memory!

Increase Vitamin C – Vitamin C is rapidly utilised by the adrenal glands in the production of all adrenal hormones (Cortisol). I recommend taking at least 3000mg per day divided up throughout the day.

Treat yourself to a massage – Getting a massage on a regular basis can help to lower your heart rate and blood pressure and promote muscle relaxation it also helps to lower your stress levels and help with the feel good factor.

Meditate – Take time out to relax and refocus your mind. As a species we do too much thinking and create stress just by what we think even if it is not true. Stress and anxiety come about by trying to predict events that may happen in the future. Meditation is a habitual process of training your mind to observe but not engage in thoughts. Allow them to flow in and out and just let them go. It can give you a sense of calm, peace and balance that can benefit both your emotional well-being and your overall health.

People also use the practice to develop other beneficial habits and feelings, such as a positive mood and outlook, self-discipline and healthy sleep patterns.

As you can see, it is vitally important to be proactive in recognising and reducing stress in our lives to remain healthy. Our bodies are designed to cope with it in small bursts to keep us alive as part of our fight or flight response, but continual stress from the numerous sources around today can affect your health.

Humans are complex beings. Things are rarely black and white. We just need to start going through the process step by step. That's why it's about improving our foods, taking pressure off the immune system and taking inflammation away. Do not underestimate how powerful and important this is.

| 17 |

Take a Deep Breath

I have so many conversations about breathing. I usually get a funny look when I say, "You don't know how to breathe." Of course everyone can breathe otherwise we would be dead. What I mean is there is a way to breathe effectively and efficiently, that allows you to energise, relax, destress and support your body structurally.

I often used to joke with my son about needs. As a kid he 'needed' everything, I am sure if you have children you have experienced that. Every time he said he needed something I reminded him we only need three things... to breathe, hydrate and nourish ourselves with good food, in that order. At which point I got the usual eye roll and a laugh.

The thing is, you can only do without food for a matter of weeks, water a matter of days and breathe for a matter of minutes.

Breathing comes first and understanding how to do it right is so powerful and is an essential addition to your THRIVE! toolbox.

The simplest of all relaxation techniques is diaphragmatic breathing, also called deep breathing, or abdominal (belly) breathing.

We are born breathing this way, taking slow, deep breaths from the belly. However, over time we learn dysfunctional breathing patterns for a variety of reasons from poor posture, trauma to stress. I believe that this begins in the classroom when we start school; sitting all day has a huge impact on how we breathe.

Stress takes a long-term toll on your breathing too. Your breath becomes shallow and short. Chances are that it is your chest that rises and falls with each breath, not your belly. The fact is that small neck muscles are used to lift the rib cage to expand your lungs, when we are stressed which takes a great effort.

Breathing is one of the most important functions requiring your attention, and unfortunately the majority of people are not even aware of the importance of diaphragmatic breathing or how to do it.

Breathing is part of the autonomic nervous system (ANS) and controls the activities of organs, glands, and various involuntary muscles, such as cardiac and smooth muscles. It is made up of two parts:

- **The sympathetic nervous system (the fight or flight response)** is involved in the stimulation of activities that prepare the body for action, such as increasing the heart rate, increasing the release of sugar from the liver into the blood, and others generally considered as fight-or-flight responses, which holds our body in a position of stress.
- **The parasympathetic nervous system (rest & digest)** activates tranquil functions, such as stimulating the secretion of saliva or digestive enzymes into the stomach to deep relaxation.

Chest breathing is not the most efficient way to breathe. Over time, your diaphragm becomes tense and abdominal muscles constricted. Your neck muscles get overused and you lose the ability to breathe deeply and naturally. Breathing this way can actually increase stress levels.

Breathing with our diaphragm allows us to become calmer and to oxygenate our blood more effectively, more efficiently, alkalising our cells and relax us.

What is a Diaphragm?

The diaphragm is a strong dome shaped muscle between the abdomen and chest. When you breathe into your diaphragm, it pushes downwards - away from the chest, causing your abdominal muscles to relax and rise. Lungs expand and allow air to be drawn in.

Here is where diaphragmatic breathing comes in. It stimulates the parasympathetic nervous system, which slows down your cardiovascular system and relaxes your muscles (whereas the sympathetic nervous system is when our bodies are in a state of fight or flight).

Diaphragmatic breathing relaxes the muscles, massages the internal organs, and allows more oxygen to flow through your body.

At first, this way of breathing may feel awkward, but once you become familiar with the technique, you will be able to reduce stress on the spot by focusing on taking a few deep breaths.

Why is breathing correctly so important?

How a person breathes has a HUGE effect on their whole system.

It influences whether pathogens make it to your lungs.

It influences how well you pump your lymphatic system to remove waste to be processed and gotten rid of.

It influences your lower back and neck stability.

Also the rate of your breathing has the ability to affect your hormone levels by influencing your blood pH and how effectively you can use the oxygen that you breathe in.

Something else to consider, unless you are exercising or have just finished exercising, you should exclusively be breathing through your nose.

This is important for a number of reasons.

Firstly, the nose acts as a filter when you breathe in and has immune cells to help stop pathogens entering your system. If you breathe through your mouth you bypass this filter and these nasties pretty much have a free pass into your lungs and then bloodstream.

Secondly, when you breathe through your nose you release nitric oxide which relaxes the airways allowing you to breathe more freely and deeply, again if you breathe through the mouth you bypass this.

If you suffer from asthma, have you noticed how much you breathe through your mouth, which is way more stressful?

When you breathe through your nose, you breathe more deeply (diaphragmatically), which pulls air deeper into the lungs where there are more blood vessels. As a result, you absorb more oxygen from the air that you breathe in and can feel more energised.

If you observe a "mouth breather" you will more likely see their chest moving much more obviously as they use accessory neck and shoulder girdle muscles to help them lift and expand their rib cage.

Chest breathing is not the most efficient way to breathe.

If you chest breathe over a long period of time, your diaphragm becomes tense and abdominal muscles constricted. You lose the ability to breathe deeply and naturally and may develop dysfunctional breathing patterns.

Breathing this way can actually increase stress levels.

Breathing with our diaphragm allows you to become calmer, oxygenating our blood more effectively, alkalising our cells and relaxing us.

Diaphragm activation is important for a number of reasons.

It helps pump waste from the lymphatic system removing unwanted pathogens that the immune system has processed. If you are a mouth and chest breather you are more likely to have a stagnant lymphatic system. A stagnant lymphatic system affects the effectiveness of the immune system, resulting in an overworked or suppressed immune.

Additionally breathing diaphragmatically helps stabilise the lower back while mouth breathing puts additional stress on the neck.

Breathing at rest should be imperceptible and you should be taking approximately 16 breaths a minute. However, breathing is a subconscious process and unfortunately it is very difficult to monitor your own because as soon as you think about it you exert conscious influence over it.

An easy, though uncomfortable, test to see whether you have a tendency to breathe through your mouth or your nose is to tape your mouth closed to see whether this creates stress for you. It should be comfortable enough to sleep like this.

If you suffer from a breathing or sinus disorder, whether it is snoring, asthma or sleep apnoea, there is a high likelihood that when you are asleep you will have a tendency to breathe through your nose.

Also, if you are producing large amounts of mucus then this is a sign that your immune system is on overdrive as mucus production is a response to trying to fight something. Excess mucus can indicate a number of things, the most common being lactose intolerance, which causes inflammation, the body's response is excess nasal mucus. It is always prudent to identify and treat the cause of the issue before you are able to reprogram yourself to breathe habitually through your nose.

Changing your breathing pattern to breathe diaphragmatically and by teaching yourself to breathe in through your nose will help start to relieve a lot of chronic stress and inflammation on your system.

In turn that means you will oxygenate more of your blood, giving you more energy, which will bring you back into the parasympathetic nervous system or rest and digest cycle, becoming calm and centred.

This can make you less susceptible to picking up infections and viruses, and can give your lower back more support taking stress off the musculature of your neck.

Diaphragmatic Breathing Technique

The procedure is very simple and effective:

Find a quiet place where you know you will not be disturbed.

1. Lie down on a flat firm surface on your back and put one hand on your stomach (just below the belly button).
2. Put your other hand on your upper chest. You should feel no movement here. The breathing should come from your diaphragm and the hand on your stomach will gently rise and fall.
3. Close your eyes and breathe in through your nose for 4 seconds, feel your stomach rise as if you are pushing you hand upwards.

1. Pause and hold that breath for 4 seconds.

2. Consciously breathe out through your mouth with pursed lips for 4 seconds. Allow yourself to get used to the feel.
3. Pause and hold for 4 seconds.
4. Repeat either for a number of breaths, a timeframe or until you feel calmer and more centred.

By using your hands in this practice you get to feel where you are breathing. Once you feel comfortable in how it feels you do not need to place your hands on your chest and stomach, just be aware of the movement.

You don't have to lie down either, you can belly breathe in a sitting position with your back straight, in fact bring awareness to breathe in this way enables you to breathe whatever you are doing.

When you become used to breathing into your diaphragm, bring your attention to the flow of your breath. Just notice the flow. Is it smooth or jerky? Make a conscious effort to smooth it out, make it flow gently and smoothly. Do not rush your breath. Be gentle. Let it flow and you will discover a rhythm to the breath.

Be patient - while "breathing" sounds like an easy thing to do - diaphragmatic breathing takes practice. Practise this breathing technique at least once a day for 5-10 minutes. If you have trouble falling asleep, practise this relaxation technique before going to sleep, you may be surprised how easily you will fall asleep. Also use this breathing whilst meditating.

In working with your breath, you will discover that altering your breath sequence changes the feelings and energy throughout your body.

You will also discover that emotional stress and constricted breathing are interconnected. As you gain control over your breath, you will gain control over your emotions.

The profound relaxation induced by diaphragmatic breathing re-establishes emotional equilibrium and frees energy for the tasks of your daily living and for healing.

Diaphragmatic Breathing is one of many techniques to help you reduce anxiety, achieve deep relaxation, relieve stress and oxygenate and energise your body effectively.

Posture Impacts Your Ability to Breathe

How often do you slouch? How often do you sit? How often do you stand? Your physical posture plays an important role in breathing. The way you hold yourself, sitting or standing is one of the major factors restricting breath.

We have been conditioned to stand as little soldiers "chest out and stomach in". As you tighten your abdominal muscles, to tighten the stomach, you restrict free flowing breathing.

I remember a physical therapist telling me about a yoga teacher who had lower back pain, which was caused by her abdominal muscles being switched off because she spent her day in lycra training clothes pulling her stomach in, This had the unfortunate effect of weakening those muscles and her lower back took over. So even fashion can affect how you breathe by wanting to look a certain way in clothes.

So whether it is fashion, sitting behind a desk, sitting in a car, slouching watching the television, all of this can contribute to unhealthy breathing patterns.

This is why breathing is so important, it alters how you feel in moments, improve your energy and lift your mood.

Try it and see.

| 18 |

The Secret to Health & Vitality

Water is the "Magic pill" everyone is searching for. I guarantee you that most people are dehydrated every day, with no real idea what being hydrated looks like. It really is the secret to health and vitality.

One of the easiest ways to improve your health and body composition is to look at what you drink or don't drink.

You would be amazed how many people tell me that they don't like the taste of water. However it is not the taste they don't like, considering it has no taste. It is the fact that so many people are so used to drinking highly sugared or flavoured drinks that their brain has "rewired" their taste buds and believe it is bland.

It's pretty much common knowledge that the adult human body is over 60% water. That means that if you weighed 80kg then 48kg of you is made up of water. That is a large amount. So it goes to show that it is vital for our health and yet so many do not drink enough.

Water is vital for our health and so making sure you give your body what it needs would allow you to function optimally.

You may be wondering why it is so important. Well I am going to tell you...

Water has 6 main functions:

Transportation

Cleaning

Reacting

Dissolving

Shock Absorption

Temperature Regulation

Let's take a closer look at these...

Transporting

As the major constitute of blood, water transports nutrients and oxygen that are important for cell growth and repair, vital messages from hormones and cell waste products such as carbon dioxide.

Cleaning

Water is used to flush toxins out of our bodies, via the skin, liver and kidneys.

Reacting

Water molecules are used in most of the body's chemical reactions. Sometimes they have to be broken down or hydrolysed to be used.

Dissolving

Water is a solvent and helps dissolve most things in the body so they can be transported round the body.

Shock Absorption

Water is an important constituent of joints and is used as a shock absorber. It prevents skeletal joints from smashing into one another when you jump, move or even fall. Water makes up the filling of your vertebral discs to allow you to jump, twist and bend without pain.

Temperature regulation

Water helps you rid your body of excess heat via sweating. Blood vessels near the skin excrete water in the form of sweat and cool the blood near the surface of the skin.

The Problem

Most people are in a state of chronic dehydration.

Often they mistake "hunger pangs" (those feelings in your stomach that most people link to hunger) for requiring food, even if they have just eaten, when in fact dehydration causes the same feeling. The sensation you feel is simply the body requiring something.

There is one thing above all else that can have a massive impact on your health, training and performance.

WATER!!

Nearly every client I have collaborated with has had sub optimal hydration when questioned in our initial meeting. They simply had no awareness of the importance of water.

The first thing I ask new clients is how much clean water they are drinking, and I mean clean water. Tea (unless it is herbal tea), coffee, energy drinks and alcohol DO NOT COUNT!

These drinks are stimulants affecting adrenal function and insulin production and can actually cause dehydration. Without even focussing on training, most people are in a state of dehydration every day, which can lead to all manner of general health issues such as:

Low back pain

Neck pain

Angina

Headaches

Depression

High blood pressure

Pain

Weight gain

Asthma

Allergies

Diabetes

So you can see immediately that if we are not sufficiently hydrated then a lot of bodily functions will simply not perform. Chronic dehydration can lead to all kinds of health issues.

Water in Performance

From a performance perspective a lack of water also affects our movement, strength and endurance, the last thing that you want to happen.

How much water is involved in critical processes?

Brain function

Water composes 75% of your brain. If your brain is dehydrated everything else is going to suffer including performance.

Blood flow

Water makes up 83% of your blood. If you are dehydrated your blood becomes thicker and your heart has to work harder not only to get nutrients to cells but to remove waste processes from the body. For example, lactic acid produced from exercise.

Temperature regulation

Your body loses water and other minerals through sweating which is vital to maintain the correct core body temperature. This is why it is so important to be hydrated before exercising and make sure you take water on board when training.

Joint health

The synovial fluid that protects your joints is made up of water. Dehydration causes aches and pains and possible injury in the joints if they are not lubricated.

Nutrient absorption

If your cells are dehydrated then it is harder for them to absorb the nutrients you need to function as their function is impaired.

Energy production

Used for digestion to move digested food through or intestines to allow us to absorb vital nutrients; if there isn't enough we will not get the nutrients we need or allow our digestive system to work properly.

Muscle Contraction

Your muscles are around 75% water which is vital for proper muscle contraction and waste disposal. If you lose even just 3% of this water causes a 10% drop in strength and an 8% loss in speed.

As well as general health issues, being dehydrated has implications for your training and how you perform.

A person is considered dehydrated if they have lost 2 percent of their bodyweight via sweating. Blood volume is heavily reliant on adequate water. If dehydration occurs and blood volume drops your body has to work harder to pump blood round the body, making it harder to get vital nutrients to our cells, especially under load such as exercise.

This may also lead to muscle cramping, fatigue, dizziness and the effects of heat stroke.

Common causes of dehydration for people who exercise in general are:

Inadequate fluid intake

Excessive sweating

Failure to replace fluid losses during and after exercise

Exercising in dry, hot weather

Drinking only when thirsty

Water intake is essential for everyone. We perspire around 500 ml of water through sweating during the night alone, so it is imperative that you start hydrating as soon as you wake.

Water for Fat Loss

Why water helps with weight loss may be obvious. If you are dehydrated your body uses signals you may mistake for hunger to get you to drink. More often than not we reach for food not water, which means more calories.

Not only does water make you feel fuller, so you eat less, drinking water also replaces energy-containing drinks like juice, soda, energy drinks and flavoured water. People on average drink over 400 kcal/day in western civilisations.

Drinking water (500 mL) before three meals a day while on a diet increases fat loss in overweight and obese individuals.

A few years back, a study found that if you drank 500 mL of water, your body would use 24% more calories for 60 minutes after drinking water. The researchers figured that this was because of changes in osmolality caused by drinking water and that your body has to expend energy to bring everything back in balance.

So before you go chasing the latest weight loss supplement or performance enhancing supplement try drinking more water.

Rule of Thumb

Although it is impossible to provide specific recommendation to individuals, as a rule of thumb for every 50lb of bodyweight you should be drinking 1 litre of water and more if you are training.

The other way is to monitor the colour of your urine. Light coloured, diluted urine probably means you are hydrated; dark coloured, concentrated urine probably means you are dehydrated.

Make sure you hydrate yourself well and ensure tap water is filtered.

And then as long as you don't have any kidney issues, maybe add a tiny pinch of pink Himalayan salt, because when you drink water, tap water is pretty devoid most good things and full of nasty things.

Increasing your water consumption causes more frequent urination. To improve absorption into the cells, it is necessary to add trace minerals such as pink Himalayan salt; this shouldn't change the taste but it can help your hydration status.

The Sports Drink Phenomenon

Whilst drinking water and hydrating through the day requires only water, when you are training there are additional factors to consider with hydration.

When we sweat we lose vital minerals from our bodies including sodium and potassium, electrolytes essential in the uptake of water into the body.

Sports drink manufacturers have been quick to jump on this and create all manner of sports drinks all marketed to replenish the body with energy and minerals etc.

Another way to convince people that it is vital to drink them.

However these drinks are vastly overrated and are not needed unless you are performing ultra-endurance events. The sugar is of poor quality and won't actually fuel your body and the minerals and extra stimulants are either not needed (again unless you are competing in ultra-endurance events) or they are in such small quantities that they make no difference and are more of a marketing gimmick.

Coconut Water

Instead of using a sports drink, consider drinking coconut water at the end of a training session.

As a natural product it is better for rehydration and electrolytes than any sports drink, for example, it is in fact an all-natural sports drink without all the sugar and artificial ingredients that are in sports drinks. The only sugars are from the coconut water itself. It is also full of magnesium and potassium, which enhances the body's ability to hydrate after intense exercise.

Water Quality

The last thing I wanted to cover is the quality of our drinking water.

In the UK, tap water is treated with a large number of chemicals in order to kill bacteria and other microorganisms. In addition, it may contain other undesirable contaminants like toxic metal salts, hormones and pesticides, or it may become contaminated by chemicals or microbes within pipes (e.g. lead, bacteria).

Here's an example of what's frequently found in tap water that we drink every day:

Chlorine, Fluorine compounds, Trihalomethanes, Cryptosporidium, salts of: arsenic, radium, aluminium, copper, lead, mercury, cadmium, barium, hormones, nitrates and pesticides.

In fact over 350 CHEMICALS have been found in UK tap water supplies. These chemicals can lead to LOTS of health issues.

So make sure you drink bottled water or better yet get a water filter, either on bench or that fits under the sink and attaches to your mains supply.

Action plan:

Drink 1 litre of clean, filtered water for every 50lb bodyweight during the day and increase it if you are exercising (add a pinch Himalayan rock salt to every litre you drink unless you have kidney issues).

Drink 500ml of water every morning with some freshly squeezed lemon juice to rehydrate and help digestion.

Drink a glass of hot water with lemon 15-20 minutes before eating your main meal to naturally boost your levels of HCL in the gut.

Drink bottled mineral water or install a water filter, there are too many chemicals left in our water that can affect our health.

Stop using sports drinks (whether you are training or not), they are not required unless you are competing in ultra endurance events. Most have poor sugar content and stimulants you don't need.

If you want energy for a strenuous strength or conditioning session, add some BCAA's to your water before and during your training session.

Hydrate with water during training and if you need to replace lost electrolytes; coconut water is a good alternative to sports drinks.

Our body tells us every day what it needs and the requirements are simply, nutrients to help us thrive. None are more important than water. It's time to start listening and supplying your body with what it needs.

| 19 |

Nourish Yourself

It goes without saying that you know what is healthy and what is not when it comes to nourishing your body. You just don't want to say it out loud. That makes it real and admitting to yourself that the chocolate or ice cream you consume every night is not the wisest thing to give a body to thrive.

Make no mistake, your lack of good nutrition will catch up with you in the end and I don't just mean the extra pounds around your middle, I mean the longer you compromise your health through poor food choices the more likely that 'disease' will come knocking.

So let's delve in a bit further and look at some principles of what constitutes a healthy meal.

The 7 Habits to Nutritional Success

Here are 7 **habits** that will help you dramatically improve your health. If you follow these 7 habits you will naturally improve your blood sugar balance, gut health, calorie control, improve your nutrient timing, when you eat and food selection.

Habit 1 - Eat Slowly and Stop at 80% Full.

Many of us eat far too quickly. This is a conditioned response to always being in a hurry so you may have to work hard at this. At each meal we expect to eat to the point of fullness.

Unfortunately this type of eating always presents challenges to leanness, performance and health - regardless of whether we choose lower quality foods or higher quality foods. That's why this habit plays such an important role in optimising your health.

The main premise of habit one is to teach you to slow down, to listen to hunger and appetite cues and to finish the eating at the right time, which usually means stopping before you have to loosen your belt.

As you notice this habit doesn't really have much to do with what you eat, but it has everything to do with HOW someone eats. This may make it the most important habit of all.

But why?

It takes around 20 minutes for your satiety mechanism to kick in. In other words, the communication between your gut to your brain and back to your gut is slow. Because of this, if you eat quickly, you're likely to eat far too much in the 20 minute time period before your brain finally says, "I'm content. You can stop eating now".

Each meal should last 15-20 minutes. Now I understand right now, you may find that difficult. So the first step is to turn off the TV, take away distractions and slow down. Create an experience. Once you have slowed your pace, you can then start to take smaller bites, chew your food completely and taste it, otherwise known as mindful eating.

A great strategy to use is to put the fork down after every couple of bites. Have a drink and a chat with your partner or family. The aim is to get you to relax and enjoy the process of eating, rather than it being something inconvenient that you rush and try to squeeze in. The interesting thing is when you begin to slow down, you naturally tend to eat fewer calories with each meal. The key is to get in better tune with your appetite signals.

Of course, if you rush through meals, you may not feel ready to slow down to 15-20 minutes each meal. That's okay. Slowing down just a little, adding just one or two minutes, or removing just one distraction can make a big difference. You can easily take a 2 minute rest mid-meal that will slow you down. If you usually eat standing up, maybe start by sitting down. If a current meal takes 4 minutes, try to make it last 5 or 6 minutes. If you generally eat while watching TV, try turning off the TV. Chew your food more. By slowing down and breaking down your food allows for easier digestion. You should be chewing 20-25 times per mouthful. Start a conversation if others are at the table. If not, become aware of your eating habits, realise there is no hurry.

In addition to helping you to eat less, slowing down allows you to gauge fullness better. With this habit, the next goal becomes to stop eating at 80% full. This can be defined as "eating until no longer hungry" instead of "eating until full." This will take some trial and error. Eating slower and short of fullness will most likely be brand new territory for you.

When you eat a 'typical' meal today, observe how you feel immediately after finishing and every hour thereafter. If you have consumed the appropriate amount that your body needs, you may feel like this:

How you should feel after eating...

Hour 0

You might still feel a little bit hungry immediately afterwards. It takes around 20 minutes for your brain to register you have eaten. If you're a fast eater, wait until the 20 minute mark before you eat more.

Hour 1

You should still feel full with no desire to eat.

Hour 2

You might start feeling a little hungry, like you could eat something but the feeling isn't overwhelming.

Hour 3

You should feel like it's time to eat a meal. On a scale of 1 to 10, where 10 is very hungry, you should feel around 7, maybe 8. It may be more or less depending on if you have exercised and your activity level. If you don't feel hungry you may have overeaten at your last meal.

Hour 4

You are really hungry. At this point you could be a 8, 9 or even 10. This is when the feeling of 'eating anything' appears. Don't allow your hunger to get to a point that you consider poor food choices.

Some additional benefits of slower eating and stopping at 80% fullness include:

- Enhanced appetite cues for the next meal, creating consistent meal timings - meaning you will eat more regularly and get a constant supply of high quality food
- Improved digestive function
- Better performance with exercise/workouts
- More time to enjoy meals
- Better sleep if you're eating before bed. Make sure your last meal is at least 2 hours before you go to sleep.

Before you move onto the next habit, you should note that this strategy is best for you if you're interested in optimising your health.

Habit 2 - Eat Protein Dense Foods with Each Meal

Eating consistent protein throughout the day is vital for keeping your blood sugar stable, hormone creation and tissue repair.

It is also very important when it comes to meal times. In fact every meal should contain some form of protein in because protein increases satiety, it slows down digestion and keeps you fuller for longer, resulting in the consumption of fewer calories.

Other benefits of eating protein include:

Protein is essential if you exercise regularly to help rebuild and repair your muscles and promotes muscle growth when strength training. It also helps your muscles heal after injury.

It also helps balance blood glucose levels which reduces craving sand late night snacking.

Protein may boost your metabolism by increasing the thermic effect of food. Your body uses more calories to digest protein.

How much do you need?

To make it easy for you, think of serving portions equal to the size of the palm of your hand. If you are a male have 2 servings, if you are female have 1 serving with every meal.

Good quality protein sources include:

- Lean Meats – e.g. Beef, Chicken, Turkey, Bison, Venison
- Fish – E.g. Salmon, Tuna, Cod, Oily Fish

- Eggs
- Dairy – Organic Greek Yoghurt
- Beans, Peas, Legumes, Nuts, Seeds
- Protein Supplements
  - Milk Based: Whey (if tolerated)
  - Plank Based: Hemp, Pea, Rice Protein

Habit 3 - Eat Vegetables with Each Meal

Vegetables are also known as nutrient dense foods. They are packed full of micro nutrients such as vitamins, minerals and antioxidants, which are involved in things such as growth, brain development, immune function and other important processes in the body that allow you to thrive. Nutrients in vegetables work synergistically to promote optimal health.

Antioxidants for example help protect the body from free radicals, unstable molecules that are produced by your metabolism and exposure to environmental pollutants which can damage tissues and organs and have been associated with certain diseases such as Alzheimer's, heart disease and cancer.

The micronutrient content of each vegetable is different, so it's best to eat a good variety in order to consume enough vitamins and minerals. Look at eating as many colourful vegetables as possible, especially, green, orange and purple, rotating them regularly to gain the most benefit.

How much do you need?

For vegetables, think of serving a portion equal to the size of your fist. If you are a male have 2 servings, if you are female have 1 serving with every meal.

Habit 4 - Eat Some Carbohydrate Dense Foods with Some Meals, (especially after training)

The best time for carbohydrates is after exerting yourself. If you have trained intensely, you will have depleted the energy stores in your body. This is when eating carbohydrates is a good idea. Carbohydrates are also known as energy dense foods, which means snacking on them all day and having them at every meal is not a good idea if you are not expending much energy. Be aware of how much you are consuming. The best way is to use a food journal and bring awareness to what you are eating over the course of a day. Be aware, any carbohydrates that are not needed by the body will be stored as fat. (See the 'blood sugar rollercoaster' chapter for more information).

How much do you need?

Think of serving a portion of carbohydrate equal to a cupped handful. If you are a male have 2 servings, if you are female have 1 serving. The best time to eat energy dense carbohydrates is after exercise and with an evening meal only on non-exercise days.

Examples:

- Rice - Jasmine, basmati are best as they are easier to digest
- Oats - Gluten free, steel milled, whole grain oats
- Quinoa
- Potatoes and sweet potatoes
- Legumes, beans and lentils
- Fruit (berries are best due to low sugar and high nutrient density)

Habit 5 - Eat Healthy Fat Dense Foods with Most Meals

Fats are essential for your health. That is why they are known as EFA's or essential fatty acids. The surfaces of each of the trillions of cells in your body need fats to function properly. Your brain is also made up of 60% fat, so you can see that low fat diets make no sense at all.

How much do you need?

To make it easy for you, think of serving equal to the size of your thumb. If you are a male have 2 servings, if you are female have 1 serving with most meals. The only time not to have fats is when you add energy dense carbohydrates to your meal after training.

Examples:

- **Saturated Fat** (1/3 of intake) - Animal fats - eggs, dairy (if tolerated), organic butter, coconut oil.
- **Monounsaturated Fat** (1/3 of intake) - Macadamias, pecans, almonds, cashews, pistachio's, tahini, hazelnuts, olives, olive oil, peanuts, peanut butter, avocado, guacamole.
- **Polyunsaturated Fat** (1/3 of intake) - Fish oil, hemp seeds, algae oils, sunflower seeds, pumpkin seeds, walnuts, flax seeds, chia seeds, brazil nuts.

Make sure with fats, you're trying to take in a balance between the three types of fat above, making sure that your intake is equal.

Habit 6 - Drink More Water

Your body uses water for many things including metabolising fats for energy, transporting nutrients in the blood, muscle contraction, energy production and nutrient absorption (see chapter on hydration). 3% dehydration can cause 10% drop in sports performance. This is why it is vital for your health to keep your intake up.

Remember that hunger could mean either food or water. The signal is the same; we are just conditioned to think we need to eat. So if you recently ate a nutritious meal and still feel peckish, make sure you are having enough water to drink.

Start your day hydrated. We sweat up to 1 pint of fluids as we sleep as your body regulates temperature. On waking drink a pint of water at room temperature adding the juice of a fresh lemon squeezed in to help aid digestion.

Hydration Timing

- Drink 1x400ml glass of clean filtered water every hour.

Hydration Amount

- Use the rule of thumb of drinking 1 litre for every 50lb you weigh per day and more if you are physically active.

Examples

- **Clean filtered water** (bottles of mineral water – preferable in a glass bottle, mains filtered water).
- **Herbal teas** (Redbush, tusli, liquorice, peppermint, chamomile). Make sure they are naturally caffeine free.

Habit 7 - Get More Rest and Recovery

Never Neglect Sleep. It is vitally important for rest and recovery and for fat loss. Your liver is most active when you sleep, which means metabolising fats and a whole host of other processes.

Lack of sleep is also something that can disrupt your health and if you are training can stop muscle gain and halt fat loss dead in its tracks. Lack of quality sleep consistently can have a real adverse effect on your overall health and wellbeing.

Imagine though, how cool would it be to grab a good, refreshing night's sleep and what it could do for you. You wouldn't need to survive on caffeine (which in excess is damaging your adrenal glands by the way), your sugar cravings would subside, and your performance in the gym would be more effective!

Sleep Timing

- Look to get yourself into bed by 10pm and asleep by 10:30pm

Sleep Amount

- Look to getting 7-8 hours of sleep per night

Basic requirements for good quality sleep

- Go to bed and get up at the same time every day
- Create a relaxing 'going to bed routine'
- Minimise light and noise by using dark curtain, eye shades and ear plugs
- Be comfortable with the right pillow and mattress

Read the chapter 'I can't get no sleep' for a more detailed view and the importance of sleep.

Why are these principles important?

These nutrition principles are designed to…

Aid your digestion

Simply put, a healthy body and mind is dependent on a healthy digestive system, you simply cannot have one without the other.

Get your gut health right, give it the nourishment it needs and you will thrive. If you don't if can impede your health and performance, whether it be at work or training. Make sure you are doing everything you can to protect your gut, by giving it good food.

Aid your liver

You can do your liver a massive favour and instead of trying to 'fix' the symptoms (effect), look at the cause and sort them out first.

There is not clear definitive time period for how long it takes an over stressed dysfunctional liver to get back to being fully functional. What is great though is that the liver is remarkable in that given the 'tools' it needs it can regenerate given the time to do so.

By removing toxins, replenishing it with vital nutrients and reinforcing it with great nutrition allows the liver to regenerate. Give your body health and see what you get in return!

Aid your Heart

Having the correct nutrition is essential for our heart, blood vessels and blood. It is vitally important that we not only look after this transportation system but nourish it, because if it is not efficient, it will affect not only our health, but our performance in sports.

Revitalising your health for your wellbeing requires total lifestyle changes and won't occur to any noticeable degree simply by doing a bit more on the cross-trainer or eating a salad every day.

Every part of health counts and is starts with good nutrition!

By using these 7 habits you will start to look and feel better. By concentrating on what you should be doing and leaving the junk behind you will have more energy, more vitality and feel more alive.

Stop the sedation with food and alcohol and realise that you CAN look and feel better. The power lies with you to make the changes and I guarantee you that if you take the steps laid out in this guide you will realise that can have the body that you want and feel on top of the world.

| 20 |

I Can't Get No Sleep

I don't know about you but there have been times when I felt like I was on a merry-go-round and I just wanted to get off. Life can feel like that too often, we create so much busyness, trying to cram in so much into to our day (usually for other people) that we sacrifice how much rest we give ourselves.

You can argue all you want but if you are stressed and overwhelmed and trying to fit too much into your day you could be sacrificing one of the most important elements of your health… SLEEP.

When was the last time you were getting 7-8 hours quality sleep consistently?

You know you need it. You also know roughly how much you should have. But are you taking responsibility for making sure you have enough? If not, why not?

The truth is, in this modern world it seems that sleep is vastly underrated. There are simply too many things to fit in...

A night out

Watching the TV

Unwinding

Having to get to work

Working late, meeting deadlines

Leisure time, kids, family

If you don't prioritise your sleep I guarantee you that it WILL catch up with you if you continue in that vain. We do more and more and trying to fit so much into our days that sleep takes a back seat and even when you grab more sleep how restful is it?

Sleep is impacted by stress, caffeine, processed foods, blood sugar roller coasters, nutrient deficiencies and meal timing to name a few.

Sleep is vital for your health!

The chances are, you are not fully aware of what sleep actually does for you and how you can maximise your immunity, health and performance. Humans are so great at putting themselves last that they wonder why they feel run down, lack energy and have that feeling of unhappiness that they cannot shake.

Having trouble sleeping, tossing and turning all night is a sure fire way to make you tired and cranky. Your whole day becomes a struggle. You need caffeine just to wake up and get through the day and you end up going to the gym for a rest rather than a training session.

Sound familiar?

Lack of sleep is also something that disrupts your physical and mental recovery cycle. If you train and exercise regularly it can stop muscle gain and halt fat loss dead in its tracks, which can have an adverse effect on your overall health and wellbeing.

The more you wake up tired, run down and reaching for coffee, the harder it will be to maintain your weight (or lose weight). Sleep is a potent regulator of not just hunger and satiety but also mood. So when you feel rubbish, you will pick sugary, refined foods and caffeine to lift your mood.

When you get around 20% of your sleep from a deep sleep state, you will wake up refreshed and excited to move your body and eat well. Imagine how cool it would be to grab a good, refreshing night's sleep and what it could do for you.

You wouldn't need to survive on caffeine (which in excess is damaging your adrenal glands by the way), your sugar cravings would subside, and your performance in the gym would improve.

Rest and recovery isn't just a simple case of climbing into your bed and closing your eyes. It's about the amount of restorative sleep per night that YOUR body requires and keeping a consistent night time routine.

Your Body Clock

Also known as your circadian rhythm, your body clock controls much of how you function as a human being. This rhythm governs your wake and sleep cycles and when it is out of balance creates havoc with your health. Poor mood, poor sleep and poor weight management are just a few of the symptoms you will see.

Most people haven't heard of the circadian rhythm and if they have just think it's about when you go to sleep and when you wake up. However, it is about a lot more than that.

When your circadian rhythm is in balance it reflects in more energy and alertness, more positive moods and generally feeling a lot better in yourself.

Three things primarily control your circadian rhythm, namely your feed/fast cycle, light and physical activity.

Your body likes routines, this is especially true for meal times. Having regular meal times creates a healthy body with more clarity of mind and quality sleep. More and more these days though, people eat up to 8 times per day if you include snacking, often with this feeding period spread over as much as 15 hours. Eating this way has a detrimental effect on your health.

Most of us do not get enough natural light. Being stuck indoors all day under artificial light has a big impact on our circadian rhythm. It's important for us to get natural light on waking for at least 20 minutes to trigger our wakefulness state. Even just looking out of a window is enough. Having limited exposure to natural light combined with the blue light from phones and TVs makes for a poor night's sleep.

Too many people are sedentary spending far too long in a seated position. Daily physical activity is important as it is a potent signal for the circadian rhythm. It's not just about the gym sessions but any activity away from the gym such as walking or playing a sport. Your body is built to move so make it move!

There are a number of important factors of sleep to aid rest and recovery and ultimately improving your overall health such as:

- Sleep stages
- Sleep benefits
- Optimising your sleep cycle

Let's break these down to see how they apply to you...

Sleep Stages

There are 4 recognised sleep stages which we go through at different times throughout the night.

Stage 1 – Is characterised by drowsiness, relaxation of all your muscles and shallow breathing. This occurs in the first ten minutes or so of the sleep cycle.

Stage 2 - Your heart rate slows and your body starts to relax in the next 10 minutes of the sleep cycle. Your body temperature starts to drop and you become unaware of what's going on around you.

Stage 3 - Rapid Eye Movement (REM) sleep. This occurs multiple times per night and is characterised by dreams due to increased brain activity and an increased heart rate.

Stage 4 - Deep sleep. The stage you must reach for as long as possible, every night.

The Benefits of Deep Sleep

Sleep is vital part to the recovery and recuperation of your body. It is not a luxury, it is essential for your mental health and wellbeing.

From a fitness perspective rest and recovery must be considered at least as important as training and nutrition for your health. You cannot hope to train intensely on a regular basis if you are not giving your body enough quality recovery time.

There's a large release of growth hormone during sleep. Growth hormone is VITAL to muscle rebuilding and repair, fat loss and indeed all round health, and is the main reason why people suffering from a lack of sleep tend to be at an unhealthy weight and struggle at the gym.

Growth hormone is released in episodic waves during your sleep, with the largest wave coming around an hour after you fall sleep.

In 2000 a study by Cauter et al, found that when deep sleep decreases from 20% of total sleep time in males under 25, to 5% in males over 35, there is a corresponding fall in human growth hormone.

This makes it particularly important for adults to pay greater attention to ensuring they maximise deep sleep as they get older if they are hoping to reduce body fat.

Lack of sleep tends to compromise your immune system and allows a greater susceptibility to colds and infections. Indirectly this will hamper your attempts to get rid of excess weight as you won't be able to train and are likely to feel a greater need to comfort eat.

Deep sleep also ensures your memory, reaction time and mental alertness remains high throughout the day, removing the need for stimulants such as caffeine to kick start your day.

Optimising Sleep

Implementing many of the following practices into your daily / nightly routine will soon allow you to feel more energetic, more alert at work and able to push through your training sessions on your way to a strong, lean, high performing body!

These tips are written in no particular order. Don't pick and choose – they will help you optimise your sleep

1. **Set your circadian rhythm** with consistent sleep / wake cycles. Go to bed and get up at the same time every day. Your weekends should not be much different otherwise you will still confuse your body.

2. **Reduce electromagnetic forces** from around you such as tablets, mobile phones, radios and televisions as these may interfere with your brain activity.

3. **Minimise light and noise** by using dark curtains, eye shades and ear plugs. Melatonin, a hormone which aids recovery and regulates our body clock is only effective in complete darkness.

4. **Get off your phone,** laptop and stop watching the TV 1 hour before bed at the latest. The blue light from these devices will block the release of the sleep hormone melatonin. Melatonin naturally rises in the evening to trigger our sleep state.

5. **Get light exposure as soon as you wake**. Light exposure in the morning can impact your sleep at night. Light is a trigger for a wakefulness state. Thus more light is better in the early part of the day; low light after dark is best as you wind down to allow melatonin to rise to help your sleep state.

6. **Don't consume caffeine after 2 pm** - Caffeine has a half life of 5-7 hours so by drinking coffee late afternoon you'll stop your body making melatonin, which will disrupt your sleep.

7. **Don't Nap after 3 pm** and keep naps to under 1 hour. Too late or too long with disrupt the daily rhythm of the body's sleep cycle.

8. **Don't drink alcohol** within 3 hours of bed. Alcohol has a sedative affect so you'll fall asleep ok but it will affect your REM sleep and deep sleep which is responsible for restoration.

9. **Avoid nicotine**. It disrupts sleep and will often cause people to wake early due to withdrawal of nicotine from your system.

10. **Minimise disruption.** Consider if supplements or medications you are taking are disrupting your sleep.

11. **Increase physical exercise**. Many people believe 3x1 hour gym sessions are enough. In fact, there are times when less is more and if necessary scaling back the gym to daily walking helps to build a resilience in the body and calms the nervous system down, before adding exercise back in.

12. **Eat meals within a 12 hour** window or less. Studies show that mitochondrial health (your cells batteries) are healthiest in a feeding window of 9-12 hours. By giving your body a chance to 'reset' helps to optimise cell health and immunity.

13. **Have consistent food times**. Having irregular meal times affects your sleep due to miss management of blood glucose. Often we think we wake up through the night thinking it was because we needed the toilet but more likely it is your blood sugar dropping, cortisol rises to mobilise energy (emergency state).

14. **Increase nutrient density** - Many people I work with are low in essential nutrients that can be gained from eating more good quality foods. Allow your body the food it requires to cover any deficiencies.

15. **Hydration** - Poor hydration leads the body into an emergency state (am I safe?). Again this will trigger cortisol to deal with the situation which will wake you up.

16. **De-stress** - Mental and emotional stress will send you into your sympathetic (fight or flight) nervous system and that will trigger cortisol, your stress hormone, which naturally rises in the morning to wake you up. Cortisol blocks melatonin and therefore affects the quality of your sleep. Using breathing techniques and journaling as a way to bring your body into the parasympathetic nervous system (rest and digest) calms your mind down.

17. **Check your HRV** (heart rate variability) Having a LOW HRV can create all sorts of issues calming the nervous system down and thus this will trigger poor sleep.

18. **Inflammation** – Having unidentified inflammation issues like bacterial, parasitic, fungal, viral and fungal infections can cause sleep disruption. In this case, it's very important make sure you get tested as this will cause disruption with your sleep.

19. **Don't fight sleep**. You will probably end up awake for a lot longer as you will enter an over tired restless state. If you are try-

ing to read and keep nodding off just go with it and put your book down.

20. **Create a relaxing 'going to bed routine'** such as a warm bath or listening to music. Avoid mental stimulation such as television and factual / exciting books within an hour of bed time.

    Perform Diaphragmatic (Belly) Breathing before bed. Put your body is a state of relaxation to allow it to wind down, switch off and recover.

    If you struggle to relax or get restless legs, consider using magnesium an hour before bed. Magnesium acts as a tremendous relaxant and also has the added bonus of being beneficial to every cell in the body and just to let you know, it is magnesium that is the key to bone health NOT calcium as most people think. If you feel restless, then definitely give this a try.

21. **Get your hours in.** Generally 8 hours of sleep works best but experiment for 1-2 weeks a time to find what works best for you. You should definitely aim for at least 7 hours.

22. **Make your evening meal 'clean'.** Eat things that are natural and nutritious and don't stress your digestive system. Stay off the heavy foods and takeaways if you want your sleep to improve; try cruciferous vegetables (broccoli, cauliflower), fish, a little rice if necessary. A good rule of thumb, if a caveman couldn't get it, then don't eat it.

Work on implementing as many as the above as possible and over time as you add more of these suggestions, you will notice dramatic differences in the quality of your sleep. I would suggest that every few weeks you add a few more of these suggestions into your routine to better make them stick.

This is the key. Whilst it is accepted that 7-8 hours is the optimal range of sleep per night, you need to pay close attention to the quality of that sleep.

Every part of health counts!

Optimise your rest and recovery and see the results of your dedication to your health. Now go and make sure you get enough sleep and reap the rewards.

| 21 |

Inflammation

I have got to say, this is one of the most misunderstood reactions in the body.

It's something that is highly likely under most people's radar. It is one of the biggest risk factors of health because virtually no one is aware it exists and yet it can have a massive impact on your life.

So what is inflammation?

The standard quote that you may relate to is…

"Inflammation is the result of an immune response to irritation, infection, or injury."

For most, inflammation is a result of turning an ankle or some form of training mishap, which is true. Short term inflammation is critical for your body's ability to protect itself. However, longer term there is another level of inflammation you probably haven't considered.

You may connect inflammation to swelling or something you can actually feel directly, however, it is low level chronic and systemic inflammation that few realise, that can have a massive impact to your health.

When we are under constant stress, the pressures of work, eating the wrong foods, working out too much, failing to get enough deep sleep and restoration, we develop a high level of inflammation that the immune system has a hard time keeping at bay, which in turn lowers our immune response as immunity has been compromised.

Where Does Inflammation Start?

Most inflammatory diseases and disorders start in the gut with an auto immune reaction to bad food choices. Every food causes some kind of inflammatory response, whether it is anti-inflammatory or pro inflammatory. The problem is though, that too many foods cause a pro inflammatory response.

As a result, we can develop gastro intestinal issues such as IBS (irritable bowel syndrome), joint pain (arthritis), and other serious diseases as the immune system becomes weaker after years and years of fighting inflammation and so no longer functions adequately.

Autoimmune issues such as arthritis come about when the immune system attacks healthy tissue, which is why what you eat plays a major factor in joint pain.

Why you should lower excess inflammation

Over time inflammation can cause the body to breakdown and make you susceptible to a myriad of diseases. Your immune system is simply overburdened and starts affecting nerves, organs, connective tissue, joints and muscles.

By lowering excess inflammation, you make your body resistant to disease such as cancer, heart disease, stroke, diabetes, Alzheimer's disease, asthma, arthritis and IBS.

This isn't to say these things will never occur, but by lowering inflammation you will be able to better bulletproof your body against them.

There are other factors too.

Our environment has a big part to play. The study of epigenetics for example suggests that our genetics are only 30% of the story, our environment makes up 70% of what happens to us. Genetics loads the gun, environment pulls the trigger.

When inflammation goes up, the body has an immune response to lower it by increasing cortisol levels, as cortisol is an anti-inflammatory hormone. This ultimately affects how your hormones work as your body then has to work hard to keep the balance.

Remember as well as a stress hormone, cortisol is part of your circadian rhythm (wake and sleep cycle) so if it is raised too often it affects your sleep, rest and recovery. It is also part of the fight or flight response so it mobilises energy into your blood stream, creating a spike in insulin as the body balances glucose.

Essential Fatty Acids

High inflammation can be due to too much Omega 6 consumption and not enough Omega 3 fats. Modern day living brings the ratio to around 1:20 omega 3 to 6 as not enough omega 3 from fish is consumed.

Omega 6 is pro-inflammatory whilst Omega 3 is anti-inflammatory. Ideally you want a 2:1 ratio of Omega 3 to 6 in your diet. This is especially important for people that are already experiencing the negatives of too much inflammation.

Why have omega 6 in your diet at all?

Our lives work on balance; our bodies go through a continuous cycle of creation and destruction every day. Our cells, continually die and renew, the cycle of life.

Omega 6 fatty acids help break down unhealthy cells that can lead to disease. If we have too much Omega 6 over a long period then we can break down healthy cells and tissues and that is where it becomes problematic.

If we take in too much Omega 3 we can have too much growth and not enough breakdown and long term this can lead to issues such as overdevelopment of potential disease.

What are some good sources of omega 3 and omega 6?

Omega 3: Flaxseed oil: chia seeds, flaxseeds, walnuts, oily Fish such as sardines and salmon, grass fed organic beef, free range organic eggs from chickens fed flaxseeds.

Omega 6: animal fats, borage oil, avocado, hempseeds, pumpkin seeds, and cashews.

In addition, adding omega 9 lowers insulin resistance, improves immune system health, and heart health.

Omega 9: olive oil, almonds, cashews, macadamia nuts, pistachios.

The Problem

So which foods cause this inflammation response in the first place and what can we do about it?

The most reactive foods studied are high sugar, grains (gluten), dairy (casein), soy and egg albumin as well as the consumption of processed foods.

For people with inflammation issues, removing the foods above for a period of time can certainly help. However, if you are not symptomatic, you might want to focus on reducing foods that are deep fried, foods that use processed oils in production and foods with highly refined flours.

Sugar plays big role in all diseases and is highly addictive. It has been suggested that sugar addiction is as bad as class a drug addiction. Ingesting so much sugar is worse than people realise and it is so easy to do because it is in so many things, even things you wouldn't think, which is why you have to read the label on everything you buy or better yet, make your meals from scratch.

To illustrate my point, have you ever tried to give up sugar for a period of time? I'm sure you will have noticed some unpleasant withdrawal symptoms.

Too much caffeine consumption also causes a lot of inflammation. Ever tried to detox from sugar and coffee? If you have you know what I am talking about. Caffeine is a stimulant that elevates cortisol which fires your stress response.

Sugar causes inflammation by prompting the hormone Insulin to be elevated all the time. Insulin is not something we want high all day long. It constricts the arteries and raises blood pressure. It causes a great deal of inflammation if left unchecked.

Grains contain pro inflammatory compounds called lectins, they also contain anti nutrients (phytates) and indigestible proteins (gluten). They often cause leaky gut (creating food intolerances) and increase inflammation in your joints.

Dairy is another factor. We cannot digest the sugar lactose, often causing excess mucus production in the nasal passages and increasing inflammation elsewhere including joints.

Gut Health

As mentioned in the 'Looking after your gut' chapter, gut health is critical for your overall health.

Along with removing reactive foods from your diet including sugar, dairy, wheat, alcohol, processed foods and caffeine, it's possible you may need supplements to maintain a healthy gut. It's always better to test than guess.

Probiotics – Can ensure that we have a good balance of healthy flora in the gut for optimal functioning and immune system health, although it's always best to understand why your gut flora is out of balance first.

Digestive enzymes – Can ensure that we extract the largest amount of energy from our food and assimilate it efficiently, again though, it's always prudent to understand what stomach acid is low or what else affects digestion, such as stress.

Two other great nutrients for decreasing gut inflammation are Ginger and glutamine. Ginger is great for any stomach issues and is a great cold fighter. Glutamine helps with healing the lining of the gut.

Other Considerations

There are a number of things you can make sure you have in your diet to help lower inflammation. Here is a list to consider...

Magnesium

Magnesium is critical for overall health and lowering inflammation. Here are some key benefits of magnesium:

Magnesium helps lower cortisol levels and drive up DHEA, which is a potent anti-inflammatory hormone.

Magnesium helps you metabolise inflammation fighting Essential Fatty Acids (EFA's).

Magnesium helps lower inflammatory responses.

Magnesium supports the adrenal glands from fatigue brought on by stress and is the ultimate stress management nutrient.

Magnesium is a vasodilator, opening up blood vessels.

Magnesium helps relax muscles.

Magnesium helps the liver to detoxify toxic chemicals.

Magnesium aids restful sleep.

Magnesium helps prevent muscle weakness and fatigue.

Zinc

Helps the body fight stress.

Has antioxidant properties.

Important for healing wounds.

Important for immune system and white cell growth.

Plays a big role in cell growth and tissue repair.

30mg-50mg of Zinc is a good daily dose. You may need more depending on how depleted you are.

Zinc Citrate or zinc gluconate absorb very well. Avoid zinc oxide which I poorly absorbed.

Vitamin C

Helps the immune system fight infection which is linked to inflammation.

Best food sources of vitamin C from food are berries (strawberries, blueberries, raspberries etc), goji berries, guavas, peppers, kale, chili peppers and broccoli.

Vitamin D

Small amounts such as 500iu has been shown to lower inflammation by 25%

Vitamin D deficiency is connected to many inflammatory related diseases: high blood pressure, diabetes, autoimmune disorders.

Important for immune system health.

Helps prevent several cancers including: bladder, breast, colon, ovarian, prostate and rectal.

3000-5000iu daily is a good dose.

Ginger

Lowers Inflammation in the large intestine.

Helps relieve stomach upset, diarrhoea, gas.

Lowers inflammation by lowering free radicals.

Effective cold and flu fighter.

Acts as a blood thinner.

Research has shown that it can reduce pain and swelling in people with Rheumatoid arthritis, osteoarthritis, and muscle pain.

Good dose is 2-4 grams is a good baseline.

Curcumin

Benefits of Curcumin include:

Found to increase detoxifying enzymes and promote healthy DNA function.

Helps support a balance between anti-inflammatory and inflammatory responses.

Acts as a free radical scavenger and antioxidant.

Curcumin molecules insert themselves into cell membranes and make the membranes more stable and orderly in a way that increases cells' resistance to infection by disease-causing microbes.

Has a positive effect on neurogenesis in the hippocampus reduction of which is associated with stress, depression, and anxiety.

Helps to block conversion of testosterone into oestrogen.

Great for gut health and as a preventative for colon cancer.

Coconut Oil

Contains medium chain fatty acids that help fight infections and organ damage.

Supports the immune system.

Fights many viral and bacterial infections.

Reduces inflammation and immune response caused by allergies.

Great for energy and conversion of cholesterol into testosterone.

7 ways to Reduce Inflammation

If you struggle with long term inflammation issues, such as gut issues, headaches, autoimmunity, skin problems or other inflammatory issues, here are 7 ways to reduce inflammation and optimise health before even thinking about things such as weight loss.

Looking at this in order of importance, you have to make sure...

1. The brain is healthy

Brain inflammation is more common than you realise. It may sound extreme but many people have issues with swallowing food, constipation and yeast issues. If you struggle with smell, taste and saliva production, these are further signs of brain dysfunction. Much of this is due to poor signalling of the brain in your parasympathetic nervous system.

2. Ensure adequate levels of stomach acid and enzymes.

As you age, stress & infections drive down stomach acid which ruins things like protein digestion. Often the people who that say 'protein makes me feel heavy' are struggling with digesting protein in this instance.

3. Gallbladder issues.

Surgeons may deem this organ non-essential, but it is there for a reason. If you are lucky to still have this, the production and flow of bile is essential to help with the breakdown of fats. With poor flow, you will become deficient in fat soluble vitamins, meaning you will struggle with sex hormone production and may develop gallstones.

4. Intestinal valve issues.

When the above is present you are at greater risk of small intestinal bacterial overgrowth (SIBO), a condition when you have a reflow of bacteria into the small intestine. If this is you, you'll find that HIGH FODMAP foods will be a real struggle for you.

5. Immune barrier (leaky gut)

Trying to fix this issue first is pointless if you don't address the above issues. You have to ensure your immune system is working well. If you are reacting to lots of foods, have skin issues, migraines and such like, calming the immune response becomes of utmost importance.

6. Gut Microbiome Diversity.

The diversity of the gut microbiome is shrinking in the western world. Low diversity is associated to more diseases than I can write here. When we eat the same meals all the time, have low fibre diets, drink alcohol in excess, don't sleep well, these all negativity effect microbiome health.

7. Chronic infections (large intestine)

Your large intestine is home to a huge array of diverse bacteria / yeast and much more. However, when we get stressed, get travel illnesses, over exercise, have a poor diet, we fail to protect ourselves from infections, both bacterial and parasitic.

There are more but I hope you can see how important it is to reduce inflammation. This is why so many people are surviving in their lives and not thriving, why their health is compromised and why so many people struggle to lose weight and keep it off.

The key to reducing inflammation is to start with what you eat and ultimately ingest. Most auto immune disorders can be traced back to increased systemic inflammation.

For most people, these changes are sufficient to greatly reduce their systemic inflammation and greatly improve their quality of life. Being mindful of this will allow you to see a reduction of auto immune symptoms and more energy day to day your training. You could also notice that you recover from your training sessions much faster and have fewer trips to the doctors.

| 22 |

Allergies, Intolerances and Sensitivities

Let's talk food related inflammation.

This is a big old, slightly complex subject, but so important. So many people really mess up the difference between intolerance, sensitivity and an allergy; they don't really understand what the differences are.

The majority of people consume too many substances that are devoid of any nutrients useful to the body. Things such as processed food, sugar loaded drinks and stimulants are consumed way too regularly and over time are all detrimental to your health as your body continually works to keep itself in balance.

Simply put, all of this is killing us slowly from the inside, most people just don't know it...yet. A bold statement? Yes it is. Yet we rationalise and justify way too much when it comes to what we eat, we look at the symptoms and reach for meds instead of looking at why the symptoms are there in the first place.

We get signs and signals every day about how the 'food' we consume affects us, but they are readily dismissed and not thought about. These signs and signals could well be down to one thing...

Food Sensitivities!

What are food sensitivities and why do they matter?

Well funny you should be thinking that, I am going to tell you.

According to Theron Randolph, known as the father of environmental medicine and clinical ecology, approximately 90% of people have some kind of allergy, intolerance or sensitivity. And 9 out of 10 of those people don't realise that their symptoms are related to the food they're eating every day. They just dismiss it as the way it is, never thinking that they could be free of it.

I experienced this first hand, it took 15 years before I found out the sinus problems I had were down to being lactose intolerant.

Food sensitivities can cause serious difficulties with your long term health and should not be ignored. I have heard from many people being told by doctors that symptoms like brain fog or a lack of energy is 'all in their head', because the tests they had come back clear. Medical science does not have all the answers. You know if something isn't right with your health regardless what a medical test may say. It might just be what you are ingesting.

If you are plagued by nagging health issues that have gone unexplained by Doctors, it simply means it is beyond their remit. Doctors know a lot about their chosen field, which is great. But when health problems fall outside of that (and they do), then consider more holistic methods.

YOUR HEALTH IS YOUR NUMBER ONE PRIORITY AND YOUR RESPONSIBILITY

It is quite possible that food sensitivities are responsible for how you feel and could be causing serious difficulties with your health, so find someone to help who can investigate with great care.

For example, the simplest method for sensitivity testing is to use a good elimination diet to remove common reactive foods from your diet completely for at least two weeks. It's often the case that there are not necessarily 'bad' foods causing issues but simply because of over consumption and over exposure.

Once you have a clean slate, you can reintroduce certain foods into your diet one at a time to see if your symptoms return. Then you can consider some good testing protocols to clear out the gut and getting it back into balance to lower inflammation. The problem with standard sensitivity tests are that they aren't good enough quality to detect the lower levels of food substances that could be causing your symptoms.

If you start to take things away and you're still not improving, then it might not actually be the food that is the genuine problem because food sensitivities can be toned down or they can be turned on, depending on the level of inflammation already present.

So what is the difference between Food Sensitivities, intolerances and Allergies?

While food allergies are an immediate, potentially life-threatening immune response to food proteins, intolerances and sensitivities trigger more subtle symptoms that may take hours or days to appear. For example, symptoms you may be tempted to dismiss such as bloating, gas, constipation, lethargy or diarrhoea are not normal at all.

Allergies

Food allergies exist when an individual's immune system reacts negatively to a food or liquid causing swelling, difficulty in breathing, wheezing, itching, rashes, flushing of the skin or even anaphylactic shock soon after eating a food.

The symptoms of food allergies normally cause a quick and obvious reaction and are potentially life threatening.

Intolerances

A food intolerance response is defined as any reproducible, toxic response to food that does not involve the immune system. Essentially it is a lack of a specific enzyme used to break down the food you are eating. This causes inflammation in the gut that affects the balance of bacteria and can lead to a variety of symptoms.

So let's take lactose intolerance as an example. Lactase is the enzyme that breaks down lactose which is the sugar in milk. From birth to five years, you produce quite a lot of lactase, after which lactase dramatically decreases.

I suffered with a lactose intolerance for 15 years before I found out what it was. I went through 2 operations with general anaesthetic in my teens to sort out the problem, which didn't work. Medics focussed on the symptoms of a constant blocked nose. When I found out about lactose intolerance whilst seeing the nutritionist about my infertility, I removed the cause (consuming dairy) and never had the problem again. Never underestimate the affect consuming foods that your body doesn't like. It always lets you know, if you read the signals.

Sensitivities

Food sensitivities exist when an individual experiences difficulty in the digestion of specific foods or certain groupings of foods. Like allergies they invoke an immune response, but are far less immediate and severe. Unlike food allergies, the symptoms of food sensitivities are not as immediate or clear. It can take anywhere from a few minutes to up to 72 hours to get any symptoms. So you may eat something on a Monday and not get symptoms until Wednesday evening.

This is why food sensitivities are complex and to a certain extent why sensitivities are both dependant on your ability to digest and break foods down. If your body becomes overburdened then the level of sensitivity may go up.

Studies have suggested that as much as 30-40% of diet induced inflammation comes from food sensitivities.

Symptoms of food sensitivities:

The symptoms associated with food sensitivities are very broad. The following are some of the major symptoms:

Dark circles under your eyes, runny nose, sour taste after eating (usually next morning on waking), brain fog, itchy eyes, itchy skin, fatigue, lethargy, needing to sleep after you have eaten; mood swings, depression, restlessness, headaches, migraines, joint pain, gas, bloating, bad breath, stubborn weight loss and indigestion.

Illnesses associated with food sensitivities:

Many illnesses experienced by children and adults are associated today with food sensitivities. There are more serious medical conditions where food sensitivities can play a primary or secondary role, which include:

Irritable Bowel Syndrome (IBS), Crohn's disease, Ulcerative Colitis, functional diarrhoea, Migraine, ADD/ADHD, Depression, Insomnia, Fibromyalgia, Asthma, Inflammatory Arthritis, Atopic dermatitis, Psoriasis, Chronic Fatigue Syndrome, Obesity, Polycystic Ovary Syndrome (PCOS).

It's really important to understand that these can have a big impact on your level of inflammation and that in turn will raise your cortisol levels creating hormonal imbalances.

Red Flags

So what should you look out for if there is no immediate response to what you eat? Well there are some common things to be aware of which may indicate sensitivities to foods. These include:

- Trying different diets frequently but still not losing weight
- Feeling puffy and bloated or have swollen joints
- You just don't feel right
- Feeling as though you have hay fever which lasts all year.
- Moodiness, brain fog and headaches
- Fatigue
- Heartburn
- Joint pain
- Acne, Eczema & Dark Circles
- Gas Bloating and Constipation

Common Causes of Food Sensitivities

Food sensitivities can be caused by many different factors. The following are a few of the major causes creating this difficulty with your health, vitality and energy.

The Food industry

The food industry is massive, from production to distribution and sales, it truly is a global trillion dollar market. Foods are often picked before they are ripe and stored in chemical gas warehouses until needed to prevent ripening. Also chemicals banned in our country are often not in the country of origin, the result being that the food we consume contain chemicals and preservatives we know are harmful to your health.

Food Additives and Preservatives

Additives are used to maintain that "fresh look" of the food we buy. This means from how long it sits on supermarket shelves to enhancing the flavour of the food, food additives involve the use of over 5000 chemicals and are used for many reasons including colouring; flavouring; preserving; thickening; emulsifying; and bleaching. Food additives were also linked by Dr Benjamin Feingold to learning and behavioural difficulties in children.

Nevertheless, the food industry has continued to increase the types and quantity of food additives used in the manufacture of food today. Chemicals are toxic to our bodies and affect our biochemistry, which in turn contributes to food sensitivities and health issues.

Parasitic Infections and Candida

Now you may not want to hear this but many people today can be seriously infected by different parasites, whether that is infections caused by bacteria and viruses or infections caused by parasites. They are all foreign invaders that can wreak havoc in our bodies. These affect the functioning of the immune system and weaken it since it tries so hard to eradicate these infections.

What makes these symptoms worse are the antibiotics people take to eliminate them. These drugs MAY get rid of the infections, but they do not discriminate between healthy good bacteria or bad bacteria. They kill everything. Our gut relies on a balance of good to bad bacteria and since antibiotics kill everything, it leaves space for another problem, candida.

Candida is a fungal infection and can spread throughout the body, into your joints, muscles, and the membrane in and around your brain, affecting you physically, mentally, and emotionally.

Infections like candida create chemical imbalances leaving you vulnerable to infectious bacteria resulting things like common colds and viruses. They can lead to suffering more uncommon types of symptoms and ailments nobody seems able to diagnose, often feeling so fatigued and listless, with swollen and painful joints and muscles.

The presence of parasites and their toxins changes the chemical system within your body so you can have a chemical imbalance. Then you begin to have difficulty digesting many different foods as well as absorbing the nutrients from the food you are eating. This is why food sensitivities are often challenging to diagnose. They increase in types and intensity and you experience poorer and poorer health.

Metal & Chemical Toxins

From the mercury from dentistry fillings and vaccinations to the heavy metals that come through our domestic water pipes, people are quite sensitive to these metals and chemicals, resulting in holding metal and chemical toxins in their bodies for many years. These poisons unbalance the inner working of your biochemistry and create serious food sensitivities, often making it difficult to digest many foods.

The Mind / Body Link

Why is the mind and body one of the causes of food sensitivities? Simple. What we eat creates the hormones our body uses that affects our behaviours. Everything is linked. The food we eat is also linked to our emotions too.

The endocrine (hormonal) system responds very differently depending on whether our emotions are loving or fearful. Whether we laugh and smile or get upset or cry, it is known that fearful thoughts create physical and mental stressors to the body and as a result deliver a hormonal cascade which affects how we behave. Our stress hormone cortisol for example can be very damaging over time if it is constantly released into our bloodstream.

Problems occur when we don't allow our emotions out. If we ignore them, they can manifest in other ways. It is proven that not addressing our emotions and keeping them buried affects our body chemistry. Too many people ignore their own feelings and look to use other means to bury them. These emotional 'blocks' cause imbalances and can lead to food sensitivities, as well as many other illnesses.

Common Food Issues

Everyone's immune system is different and just because someone is allergic or sensitive to a food, doesn't mean everyone is. More often there is one food that can cause the problem, but others simply add to the toxic load. Find the cause and eliminate all the symptoms.

The main culprits that are associated with the most common food sensitivities are:

Wheat gluten, dairy, eggs, soy, shellfish, tree nuts

However other foods that are known to create sensitivities include bananas, peanuts, yogurt, kidney beans, brewers and baker's yeast. If you react to one or more of these foods, it will be a bit of an adjustment (because changing anything seems overwhelming at first) but it is absolutely possible that you can eliminate one or more of these from your diet without ever missing them to help lower inflammation.

How can I develop a healthy diet?

The first thing to do is follow the principles in the Nourish Yourself chapter. Better quality sleep, nourishing foods, good hydration. But there are other things to consider:

1. **Avoid foods to which you are intolerant and/or allergic.** First and foremost, get in tune with your own body and find out what foods are toxic to your body. Food sensitivities are very individual. You can be sensitive to a food that no one else

you know finds problematic. If you are experiencing significant symptoms, you should consider talking with a reputable health-care practitioner about your diet and suspected food sensitivities.

2. **Eat organically grown foods whenever possible.** If food sensitivities are suspected then you should avoid foods with pesticides, artificial colourings and preservatives as much as possible. Synthetic food additives are notorious for causing food sensitivities. Avoiding these artificial additives is essential in developing a diet that promotes your optimal health.

3. **Support healthy digestion**. It is important to have a fully functional digestive system. From the saliva in your mouth, to stomach acid and enzymes further down the chain, every step has to do its job. After chewing, the food's next stop is the stomach, where an adequate amount of stomach acid is needed for the breakdown of proteins. Without proper breakdown, all proteins are potential toxic food molecules, which can cause sensitivities. Low stomach acid is common and various factors can inhibit sufficient stomach acid production including pathogenic bacteria, and frequent use of antacids. If necessary, these digestive factors can be replaced with appropriate supplementation. Digestive enzyme support can also be obtained from fresh pineapple or papaya, which contain the enzyme bromelain, and other fresh vegetables and herbs.

4. **Support the gastrointestinal barrier.** The gastrointestinal cell wall is the barrier between potentially toxic food molecules and the inside of your body; the integrity of this barrier is vital to your health. Support for the cell barrier in the gastrointestinal tract is very important, especially in the stomach. The mucous layer is one way the stomach protects itself against the damaging effects of stomach acid. Alcohol, over-the-counter anti-inflammatory drugs (e.g., aspirin or ibruprophen), and pathogenic bacteria can all reduce the mucous layer, leading to lesions in the stomach. This must be protected. Choline provides nutritional

support for a healthy mucous layer and is found in vegetables such as cauliflower, lettuce and also eggs. Some foods also help combat or protect against the damage of pathogenic bacteria; these include, carotenoids found in vegetables, and vitamin C, found in many fruits and vegetables.

We are all entitled to vibrant health. With a little detective work and experimentation, you can easily find out what foods are not supportive to you, and eliminate them to start improving your health immediately.

Food sensitivities can be a minefield. The majority of people don't even realise that they are affected. However, if you just tune into your body and listen to what it is saying, eventually you will be able to be more intuitive with your nutrition because you'll learn the subtleties of how foods affect you. Food sensitivities can make a big difference to you and is probably one of the key missing elements of how you can drastically improve your health fast.

If you don't "feel" right, or if you have unexplained symptoms then seek help. If the medical profession cannot explain them that doesn't mean they doesn't exist. You know when you don't feel yourself, so start tuning into your body and seek out a health practitioner, such as a naturopath or nutritionist who can help you.

Truly knowing and understanding how your own body functions best is one of the greatest gifts you can give yourself because it's the most empowering way to achieve lasting health and well-being.

PART III – EMOTIONAL WELLBEING

| 23 |

There Are No Words

What you come to realise is that when humans are triggered emotionally, the reaction comes from the limbic system. The emotional centre of the brain doesn't speak with words but expresses itself through feelings; sensations that we interpret into thoughts and words as we try and make sense of them.

Sometimes though, we can label these sensations incorrectly, creating a narrative that can far too often leave us in the wrong part of our brain. When I say wrong part of the brain, I mean we react as part of the fight or flight response to keep us from danger.

Everyday stresses can keep us in our reactive brains which quite often create irrational and emotive decision making. This also keeps us in survival mode, unable to be creative or have clarity on who we are. When we are fighting for our survival nothing else matters. We have tunnel vision and become almost selfish with our approach to life. Hardly a way to THRIVE!

At any moment we have a choice, whether to keep being reactive or to stop, breathe and respond differently by addressing these behaviours. This starts when you start listening to your heart. When you feel what your intuition is saying before your mind gets in the way.

I Don't Trust You

When I was 3 years old I was in hospital to get my tonsils removed. Little did I know that in that moment, I would experience am overwhelming traumatic experience that would affect me throughout my whole life. I knew the story of course, I was there. I just didn't connect the dots. It wasn't until I spoke to a coaching friend of mine in 2016 that I realised. I have vivid memories of that time, being in a cot, crying as my mam left me. Climbing out of that said cot as I had wet the bed looking for someone to help me and the black mask as it descended over my face to put me to sleep.

As an adult I knew this story, my mam had recounted it many times. She didn't want to leave me, she left in tears as they told her she couldn't stay with me. How my mam was already in the hospital car park when she rang from a call box (remember those?) to see if she could come and collect me. But as a 3 year old boy, watching his mam leave him in pain all alone; that was traumatic. The person who I loved the most in the word was abandoning me. In that moment was instilled a belief that people could not be trusted, especially those that you love. Whether that was true was irrelevant, that was my truth in that moment as I cried, tears streaming down my face as my mam left the room.

When I recounted these memories and images to my friend I broke down and sobbed uncontrollably for 10 whole minutes, snot bubbles the lot. I think I ran out of tears. When I stopped blubbing an incredible thing happened. An intense energy release, starting from my stomach, the ball of light rose slowly before exiting from the top of my head. I immediately felt a lot lighter.

I realised so many things in that experience. How I unconsciously believed that those I loved the most would abandon me, so I went out of my way to prove that belief true. I created situations to push those I loved away from me to protect myself and prove I was right. Thankfully for me, those people we more stubborn that I was and stuck around, I know now how fortunate I am to have those people in my life.

| 24 |

Feeling is Healing

It is often believed that people view what holds them back as a mind-set problem, or a problem in the way they think. However I invite you to consider that mind-set does not come into it. Mind-set is a function of the neocortex, the logical, thinking part of the brain that we get to access when we are calm and centred.

When we are stressed or when we react to some form of trigger, the brain shuts down the neocortex so you are literally out of your mind. The brain doesn't want you to think about whether you are safe or in danger as this wastes potentially lifesaving moments of time. It wants you to react and do what you did the last time this happened. That is, whatever you have, 'fired and wired' in your mind to take you away from danger and towards safety.

This is why so many of us go round in circles in times of stress. Looking at the brain at a much lower level leads to the feeling system.

Thought Feeling Loop

Thoughts which appear to be driving the unwanted behaviours are themselves driven by the feeling system, in particular unresolved emotional trauma. When we try to understand whatever is showing up in our world, we create stories and belief systems in line with our past experiences. We then look for the evidence to confirm those beliefs and stories which all combines to form our identity which we eventuality physically embody and it becomes our way of being.

The acceptance of this reality leads us to learn to live within the limitations of our own unique version of the world, our personal jail if you will; a jail that we can't see, smell or touch because it's buried deep in our unconscious programming.

We may not be able to see this jail or be aware of the mind forged manacles we have created, but we can usually notice its limiting effects of it. Deep down I think we all get a sense that we are held back in some way, some sense of foreboding we ignore, but cannot shake.

We just don't know what to do to set ourselves free.

Understanding the thought feeling loop and how it influences and drives us in our beliefs and behaviours unconsciously, was the missing link for me to understand why humans often feel stuck in a loop with no way out, including me. The thing is, we can escape this mind prison we often find ourselves in, if we have the courage to do it.

| 25 |

Faulty Installation

So let's think for a moment about how we allow these traumatic experiences to influence and shape our world.

First, trauma is introduced into the system anytime we experience overwhelming experiences in life. Left unresolved they are stored and start to influence the way we think and feel. This leads to the trauma over-sensitising the amygdala (part of the limbic system responsible for controlling our emotional responses) forcing us to live in our emotional brain and therefore feeling emotionally unsafe.

We then tend to seek ways to numb out, distract or sedate ourselves in a variety of ways to avoid that unsafe feeling. As a result of this distorted perception of the world, we create all kinds of stories and beliefs to 'protect us' from danger.

When we talk about the amygdala being over sensitised, it is more commonly known as the Amygdala Hijack.

Coined by Daniel Goleman's book 'Emotional Intelligence: Why It Can Matter More Than IQ'. Amygdala Hijack is a term used to describe emotional responses from people which are immediate and overwhelming, and are usually an overreaction to the actual stimulus which has triggered a much more significant emotional threat.

Physiology Trumps Psychology

Imagine information streaming in through our sensory systems that passes up the spinal cord, then filtering through the amygdala in the limbic system. The amygdala constantly posing the question... **Am I safe?**

If everything feels predictable and familiar, the limbic system passes the information through to the neocortex, the thinking, logical brain and everything is fine.

However, if the amygdala senses that something isn't safe, it stops the information flowing to the neocortex immediately and mobilises the fight, flight or freeze response in the autonomic nervous system. We are not allowed to think, only react and do whatever programs or beliefs we installed the last time that kept us safe.

If you have ever felt nervous you will recognise the familiar feelings of fear, stress, anxiety, anger and sickness. Our ability to think rationally is impaired and access to our higher cognitive functions such as reasoning, decision making, planning and inhibition are downregulated.

At best this takes away our ability to deal with the situation powerfully, and at worst we can end up doing all kind of things that we didn't intend to do, and later regret. We are literally out of our minds as the amygdala refuses access.

| 26 |

Releasing Emotions

We are hardwired to move away from pain. It sounds counter intuitive, but to allow you to fully resolve any traumatic, emotional pain from past or present that is influencing your life in a negative way, the basis of the emotional release system is training you to feel safe whilst you do the exact opposite to what you are deeply wired to do, which is to move away from pain.

When you are growing up as a child and exploring the world, you soon learn that when physically something hurts, you move away from it. Whether it was falling off your bike, trapping your fingers, cutting yourself, burning yourself or causing yourself pain in some other way, you quickly learn strategies to avoid doing such things, I know I did. From falling from a quarry wall (don't ask) to going over the handlebars on my bike, I definitely remember thinking I am NOT doing that again!

When you start developing emotionally, the exact same strategy is employed; when something hurts you move away from it. However, when it comes to the emotional realm, you need to complete the feeling level aspect of the experience, otherwise you take it in and store it in your emotional system, creating an 'emotional splinter'. Imagine a wooden splinter in your finger that you do not remove. Over time the pain fades, however, any time you catch the exact point the wooden splinter entered, it reminds you it is there with an ache or even sharp pain. That will continue until you remove it. It is the same with unresolved emotional trauma. If the emotional pain is not resolved, it's that exact process that over-sensitises the Amygdala and causes all the problems.

So by SAFELY going into your emotional/feeling system and allowing yourself to complete the incomplete, feeling level experiences, you truly let them go. In the process, the Amygdala will downregulate and calm down, stopping the war within and replacing it with peace by gaining freedom from disempowering thoughts.

Human Needs Alignment

If we look at the classic - Maslow's Hierarchy of Human Needs we can take a different view of creating a healing framework to help you understand how to build safety by strengthening your emotional resilience. See how by satisfying our basic foundational needs it allows us to access higher level feel good and achievement needs allowing the development of an amazing healing framework:

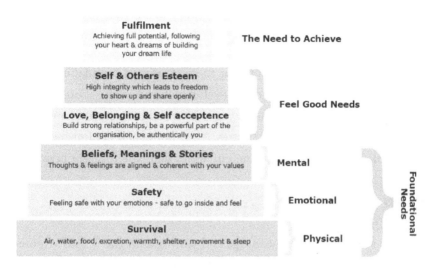

Human Needs Alignment
Image courtesy of Rise & Shine

Having worked with hundreds of people, I found that humans are prone to working on the exciting things in life, like chasing our dreams, achieving goals, creating our dream business, increasing our income. Now these things are really cool things to aim for, but unless you build solid physical, mental and emotional foundations first, you are unlikely to succeed.

So what do I mean by foundations?

The need to achieve comes in the fulfilment section at the top of the pyramid in the human needs diagram. Now that is fine as long as the support structure below that is strong. Fulfilment requires everything below it to be sturdy and fully supported. If not, you run a real risk of crashing emotionally and being frustrated at not being able to take the actions required to achieve your goal.

How often have you set goals only for them to come crashing down when in a stressful state triggered by some emotional event? If the brain doesn't feel safe, the Amygdala highjacks your normal flow and shuts off your logical brain and gets you to react and do what you did the last time to keep you safe, even if consciously it wasn't what you desired.

Based on this framework, building solid emotional foundations starts by making sure the need at each level is met and is the stronger for it from the bottom up. This leaves you with a solid structure from which to build whatever your heart desires. Your hopes and dreams feel more achievable as you feel safe to open up more than you thought possible.

Who Am I?

We can rewrite beliefs, meanings and stories with the "I AM" framework. It's common when asking for help to address past trauma, to actually revisit that trauma. In my experience, this is one thing I feel is of little benefit because talking about past experiences over and over without allowing the body to release the energy around that trauma, makes the person focus and relive the event as if it is happening again and again.

The 'I AM' framework allows you to shift belief systems quickly and without having to know what created the belief in the first place.

I AM are two of the most powerful words you have in your vocabulary because the words which follow shape your reality.

The key to creating a new personal reality is by aligning with your 'I AM' statement and actually feeling it, rather than just thinking or saying it.

For example if you say 'I am healthy', listen to your body's response. Scan your body from your head to your toes as you say the phrase. What sensations do you feel? Do you contract or expand? Does your energy go up or down? Do you feel unhealthy? Do you feel guilt or shame? Or do you feel elevated with joy?

Saying the statement and feeling where your energy is in your body lets you know whether you believe the statement. If the feeling is heavy or uncomfortable, as much as you want to believe it you don't as your body is highlighting an 'emotional splinter'; a past trauma that has not been fully felt or cleared. That's when you get to be with that feeling, fully feel it and let it go.

Our bodies are so intelligent the more we listen, feel fully and connect with the 'I AM' the freer we are to experience the life on a whole new level.

Letting Go

Having worked with so many people, I believe being able to let go of emotional trauma is one of the most powerful things we can do. By tuning into and listening to your body removes stories and beliefs created to keep you 'safe', even to the expense of those beliefs holding you back. Once you allow yourself to full feel these repressed experiences your brain will have no more use for the stories keeping you safe from that trauma and lets them go too.

I have seen many people have visions, visual representations of what the link was between the repressed emotions and why it happened. Others, have an overwhelming surge of energy being released, which I have experienced. Some people have realisations of past events that they never even contemplated.

When we create unconscious behaviours we don't see the correlation to past events. We carry stores and beliefs around guilt and shame and rejection. We store emotions such as anger to project us away from the real issues deemed too painful by the brain because of the experience that created them.

Allowing yourself to let go and release the energy lightens the load. You regain part of yourself you may not have realised you had lost. It is akin to a veil being lifted that allows you to see the truth.

If we don't allow ourselves to be fully heard, seen and felt, we can create a world where we are almost looking down from above. An off the cuff remark caught in an emotional state can allow us to shrink as we become emotionally 'stunted'. Releasing these internal self-limiting emotions around these experiences will set you free.

| 27 |

Express Yourself

Our brain is constantly asking 'Am I safe?' You may have noticed by now that this is a theme running throughout this book. Allowing the brain to feel safe moves us up the human needs hierarchy. Get the foundations solid and we have a better base with which to build emotional resilience allowing us to thrive.

Emotional pain can be very unpleasant and as a result we will unconsciously move away from it; our brain's way of protecting itself. We all experience painful emotions, which can be traced to things that have happened to us though our past experiences.

Unresolved painful emotions are deemed unsafe and so we create a belief, story or narrative to take us away from that pain, which as I mentioned at the beginning of the chapter becomes part of our world view or identity. I invite you to consider that by understanding that your limbic system simply wants a voice to express itself, to be seen and heard; to be felt. It wants recognition of the feelings that it uses to communicate with you. It wants you to full feel, resolve and let go of painful emotions. By doing so it can change how you think, what you believe, the fears you have, the emotional blocks that can often keep you stuck.

This for me and all of my clients is a game changer.

PART IV – MENTAL FITNESS

| 28 |

Mental Stigmas

Mental health still carries a stigma to the uneducated and uninitiated. There is way more awareness of mental health nowadays but I still see people, especially men, who suffer in silence. That is why I work with men to help them unburden their deep rooted beliefs around shame and help remove internal self-limiting emotions that influence their world view.

When Joy became pregnant way back in 2004, mental health was rarely talked about. It certainly wasn't mainstream and it was what happened to 'other' people. It was steeped in shame and buried feelings. It was about 'crazy' people and I remember how it was shied away from.

I had encountered mental illness in my teens with my mam, I didn't really understand it back then, but knew my mam was suffering and I couldn't do anything about it. So I kind of just got on with life. I was too young to understand, but I do remember being frustrated that I couldn't help her. There were times when she was so medicated that she didn't know where she was. I remember thinking, "I do not want to be like that". It was around that time that my perception of exercise and looking after myself changed. I was determined never to be that way.

It's not until you have first-hand experience of mental health that your eyes get opened.

When Joy became pregnant naturally after so many years of trying, we were elated, our own miracle. We looked forward to enjoying the pregnancy after so long trying. But it soon became apparent there was to be another twist to the story and not in the way we ever expected.

It started soon after we discovered Joy was pregnant.

Nausea.

For the longest time we thought it was morning sickness, that shift in hormones that so many women encounter when they first become pregnant. But Joy's persisted, it was making her really ill. We tried everything, the traditional and the not so traditional methods to quell the sensations. But nothing really worked. It wasn't until the consultant at the hospital prescribed the most powerful anti-nausea medication you can take which didn't make any difference that the penny finally dropped.

It wasn't morning sickness at all, it was crippling anxiety.

From the moment Joy became pregnant, this incredibly happy moment was also the trigger for something she was unaware of. What we expected to be the happiest time of our lives turned out to be the complete opposite.

I can safely say that the pregnancy was bittersweet. Having tried for so long to conceive, then beating the odds and confounding the medics by conceiving naturally, what came next was harrowing and painful. No one likes to watch their loved ones suffer. I was to watch on helplessly as Joy suffered during the whole of her pregnancy and beyond.

Joy ended up in hospital for 5 months and I stopped work to be there to support her every day. I had my own business which helped, but if wasn't for the support from our parents it would have been a lot harder.

I haven't really thought about this for a long time. I have realised whilst writing about it I still have unresolved energy and emotions around how I felt back then as I cast my mind back and unlock those memories. Now I have the tools to process these unexpected feelings, but back then I was lost, so I did what so many blokes would do, I locked them away and I buried them deep.

On the outside, I was visiting and supporting Joy every day. On the inside, I stopped living. I pushed my emotions way down to help me cope with the pain. I closed my heart. I didn't want to feel that hurt anymore. I made a choice to be there for Joy. There were days when I returned home feeling shell shocked; tears streaming down my face. I remember driving home with no memory of the journey. I would get home and stare at the walls. Time slipped by and when I woke up it felt like Groundhog Day… reliving the same nightmare again and again. Watching your wife suffer isn't something I would wish on anyone.

But the feeling of helplessness didn't sit well with me. How could I help her? I poured over nutrition books, books on fear and anxiety and trauma, I contacted holistic health practitioners, hypnotists, homeopaths and faith healers. I wanted to take Joy's pain away, not realising how much pain I too was feeling.

The thing is, I couldn't 'fix' Joy. I could only try and understand what was going on and support her, but at the time I didn't know any different. As a result I suffered in silence and I didn't open up to anyone.

One thing I have since realised is that you have to put yourself first. There is no point in running yourself ragged for someone else if you haven't took time for your own 'self-care', recharging your own batteries so you are in a better position help others. If you are putting yourself down the pecking order you will become unstuck eventually. You will be tired, burnt out, maybe even feeling depressed and anxious. You cannot help anyone from that place. By putting yourself first, you energise yourself so you have the energy to help others. It's better to start with 100% energy by taking some time out for you first rather than starting at 30%. You cannot help anyone when you are running on empty.

| 29 |

Worrying About the Future

Did you know that humans are the only species on this planet that frequently think about the future? As a result, this creates an unpleasant feeling as the brain feels unsafe, not knowing what is going to happen. The unpleasant feeling is anxiety.

Why?

Anxiety can take many forms for many reasons. In essence, anxiety is focusing on something that the brain cannot predict a response to. It is impossible to know what is going to happen in the future and yet humans try and predict it all the time. Your brain likes to know what is going to happen and when it can't it senses threat, which triggers your fight or flight response.

When you allow fear to trigger you over and over and do nothing about it, it can create a negative impact on your life. Being stuck in a loop can result in a downward spiral. If you have experienced any kind of anxiety in your life you might just relate.

Experiencing the destructive power of anxiety can be terrifying even if you know the biological processes involved. It can be all consuming. I have witnessed the terror and all-consuming fear in others close to me and I have experienced it myself. I have cowered in a corner, curled up in a ball, afraid to face the world. Let's just say it's not pleasant. Regardless of the severity, it is always very real to the person experiencing it.

Your brain is the ultimate survival machine. It doesn't care how you feel as long as you are alive, although you might beg to differ if you have ever suffered from long term anxiety before.

Being a coach I have studied anxiety in depth. I have worked with people with acute anxiety, bipolar disorder and manic depression very successfully. I know when you are in that hole, that dark place seems inescapable, when fear grips you so tight you want your world to end. You think, there is no way out. It feels too scary (unsafe) to contemplate. Sometimes though, when you find the courage, there are people to help. You may think you are alone until someone jumps into that hole with you and says 'I have been here before and I know the way out'.

Let's be clear though. You do not catch anxiety. It is a state fuelled by overwhelming emotional response to not feeling safe.

Once you realise this, you can take back control of your life if you choose to. Hiding behind the label of anxiety only ever keeps you in a victim state. I don't say this flippantly, I know how bad anxiety can feel. Anxiety can be exacerbated by chemical imbalances and are a result of things such as poor nutrition, toxicity and excess cortisol from constantly projecting thoughts into the future. Quite often these thoughts are a result of repressed or unprocessed emotions.

These feelings drive us to become imbalanced and many people believe they cannot overcome anxiety and yet I have worked with hundreds of people and know you can move past this. You can resolve the deeper drivers driving anxiety by downregulating the nervous system and by resolving/removing the fearful projections that are stored deep in your unconscious mind. Unless you are open to look at the deeper issues and make the difficult choices and do something that changes your focus and state you will remain stuck.

You can look at anxiety in two ways. Short term 'conscious' anxiety; when there is an expectation of something new or near into the future. Chronic, long term 'unconscious' anxiety is driven from unresolved, unconscious internal beliefs from sometime in your past.

Conscious anxiety

This usually occurs when something new is presented to you that is happening in the near future; a new venture, a new job, or a new exercise class. It could be standing in front of an audience for the first time or going to a new country. Maybe you are going to jump out of a plane or bungee jump or it could be a physical altercation. Until you have experienced it at least once, you will feel nervous and have those feelings we attach to it, when in fact it's a perfectly normal response to what we label fear, the fight or flight response, to keep us safe. The only way to desensitising this sensation is to face it and remove what the brain deems a threat by demonstrating that it isn't.

But what happens when it feels disproportionate to the situation?

Unconscious Anxiety

There is always a reason for anxiety to be triggered, most often though, it is unconscious. I have worked with people who had unexplained anxiety that turned out to be an object in a room of their house from an ex-husband who physically abused them. I have worked with someone with debilitating claustrophobia because they were made to watch a horror film as a kid and then locked in a cupboard. I have worked with someone so angry at the world because of an abusive childhood and used anger to mask the pain.

There are times when you don't know why you feel anxiety, or the trigger that sets it off. An unconscious belief from an overwhelming traumatic experience trapped in the body will create that feeling of being unsafe. Sometimes the brain can feel so threatened that anxiety can be crippling. Childhood trauma can feel so unsafe it can perpetuate through your entire life, literally altering your view of the world. (see Part 3: Emotional Wellbeing for more)

Are you listening?

Our body gives us the opportunity to confront our deepest fears or traumas, it depends whether we are paying attention. Subtle signs, signals and behaviours present themselves as warning bells, but often go unheard. Trauma creates disconnection as we unconsciously move away from pain. We build stories and beliefs to keep us safe and away from that pain, which can cause anxiety, we just don't know why because we don't connect the dots. Eventually though the universe makes us pay attention, the lessons get louder and louder until they cannot be ignored.

You get to choose whether to be a victim or a victor. No matter how bad it feels and whatever is behind it there is still a choice to be made. Amidst the category 5 hurricane of your own making there is peace. The eyewall of the storm, a centre where you can observe instead of engage, where you can be calm and centred as the chaos around you ensues and consumes. Yes it feels scary as hell, but if you are courageous, you can choose differently and let the story around anxiety go.

| 30 |

Three Brains? Really?

Our brains are a marvel; did you know there are three parts of your brain all working seamlessly together? Understanding how they work in synergy will show you (I hope) why in times of stress humans do the things they do, often it seems against their will.

The three regions are the reptilian brain also known as the basal ganglia, the mammalian brain also known as the limbic system and the human brain or neocortex.

The reptilian brain is in charge of your primal instincts such as the fight or flight response, the limbic system controls our emotions and the neocortex is responsible for logic, creativity and rational thinking.

You see, the human triune brain is very clever. It is constantly looking to keep you safe (I may have mentioned that once or twice, throughout this book!). It wants to survive and so the reptilian brain in times of threat prepares us to fight or flee.

The amygdala (part of the limbic system) in the brain is constantly looking to see if you are safe. Any form of stress/threat is instantly upregulated and the neocortex (thinking / logical brain) downregulated so in times of 'danger' you are not allowed to think, you react and do what you did the last time to keep you safe. Why are you not allowed to think? Because in times of threat the neocortex is too slow to make a decision that could be potentially life threatening.

Back in the caveman days your brain didn't want you to spend time thinking about whether to run from the wild animal fast approaching you, it wanted you to react and do what you did the last time you faced that danger to survive.

There is no danger of sabre toothed tigers these days; that has been replaced by every day stresses of modern life. These stresses are deemed unsafe by your brain and so you react and do what you have fired and wired your brain to do in these situations.

At some point in your life you have programmed the brain to do something specific in certain stressful or threatening situations. That can be anything such as alcohol, drugs, food, gambling or anything to take you away from the immediate pain you are facing.

Each time a trigger arises you automatically reach for whatever you have 'deemed safe'.

For example, have you ever had a 'bad day' at work come home and reached for a bottle of wine or some chocolate. Maybe you are trying to lose some weight or trying to be healthier. After the 'event' you may feel guilt or berate yourself for being weak willed. The thing is you did exactly what you programmed your mind to do in times of stress. In reality you were literally out of your mind!

Here's the revelation, it's not in the mind… it is all in the brain. Physiology trumps psychology only 100% of the time. It's hardwired by design to keep us safe.

I think it's important to understand ourselves more, how we react and how we feel in certain situation. Bringing awareness to this is the first step to allow us to change it if it doesn't serve us. We are unique, every single day. There is only one of you, just like there is only one of me. Every single day we wake up a different person. We have different stresses, food, hormones, sleep quality/quantity and hydration levels and therefore we are slightly different EVERYDAY.

Consider that we are a combination of two things, instinct and experience. Your unique reaction to a person, situation or circumstance is very much driven from our base instincts that have remained in us from our caveman days. The survival instinct is life saving and the brain is the ultimate survival machine. It remains strong within us and will drive us to act in certain ways depending on the level of threat.

Laid on top of this are our own experiences that are hardwired into us. These two combined, the base human instincts and our stories that we store, give our life predictability. We also all have our own value system that we have built from our experiences. These are the things that give us an instant reaction to something when we think or see them.

But what does this mean?

Well they are some key things you get to realise to succeed in having a thriving life. It's not in YOUR mind, it's in your brain; it is how you have programmed it to react.

With that in mind, here are some ways how to understand how your brain works and how you can create a thriving life:

Predicting a response

Based on our survival instinct our brain will look for patterns that it can predict as "safe" even if they are not in our best interests.

E.g. the bottle of wine after a bad day.

Action: List out the first thing you will change to improve your life in some way. How will you start it? How will you measure it? Who will support you?

The brain fears change

The brain wants to protect you and keep you alive at all costs. Remember, when you are feeling fear the thinking part of your brain is switched off and we cannot use it. Our survival system wants us to react and do what we did the last time. We will act on past stories and experiences to keep us safe.

Action: Question your beliefs. E.g. 'I've had a hard day, I deserve a treat or a glass of wine'. Ask 'does it serve my purpose?'. Beware of moral licence and justifying your behaviours with 'need', 'deserve', 'treat' or 'reward'. Be mindful of these hard wired justifications. Did you really earn that bottle of wine after a hard day at work?

Fired and wired

We are human, our brains are wired to work in a certain way. We evolved from cavemen where our fears were based on staying alive, eating and sleeping. Nothing has changed at a primal level hence we like predictability and stories. The fired and wired emotions lead to actions. 'I've had a hard day' equals 'I deserve a bottle of wine', remember?

Action: Challenge these fired and wired links, ask yourself every time 'does it serve my purpose?' or 'is it true?'. 'If I drink that wine does it serve my purpose?', 'Is it true it makes me a failure?'

You will fear change

The feeling of fear can be triggered by a change that was too fast, too slow or something the brain is not sure of the intent. The reactions to fear can include fight, flight or freeze. Remember, when feeling fear you can't use the thinking part of your brain, you revert to past experiences and stories.

Action: Recognise your fears and verbalise them to make them less of a threat. Get it out of your head and face it down. Be aware of fear in others and try not to judge. E.g. is your partner being argumentative when you get home from work? What are they reacting to? What can you help them with? Being more aware in this way will make you less judgemental.

Wired for Negativity

Because our brain is the ultimate survival machine, it is hyper vigilant and will cling to the negative as it is more likely to endanger us. It will also err on the side of caution to give us the best chance of survival.

Action: Challenge your negative thoughts by asking 'Is that true?', challenge your truth and be mindful of the meaning you are attaching to the words you use.

Speed of change

We all have a reaction to the speed of change. E.g. for some it can be fast for others it has to be slower. Think about your own reactions and how you cope with change. We always get to choose the next step that feels good for us. If we go too fast, or too slow or if we freeze, that stimulates our stress response and we will have that strong urge to react and do what we did the last time in that situation.

Action: Put in place small steps to change. E.g. if you are embarking on a new healthy lifestyle, pick one or two things to change and action them at your own pace. It's easy to get caught up in what everyone else is doing or how fast they did it. Consider that comparison is the thief of all joy, focus on yourself and take it at your pace.

Self-esteem bank

Reward yourself and value what you have achieved. Your energy goes where your focus goes, make sure it is on something positive. Our brain has a goal seeking hormone called dopamine which drives us onto a goal no matter what is in the way and measures our success only against that goal. However when we reach that goal it doesn't reward us with a virtual thank you. Like a torpedo it looks for its next target.

Action: Reward yourself for the small steps you take towards a goal. Take time to count your wins, write them down in a journal, recognise them and pat yourself on the back for what you have done at the end of each day. Get that happy hormone fix. Think of it as adding to the self-esteem bank account, you get to keep the promises you made to yourself by doing what you said you would. Each time you take a step towards a goal add a credit. The more credits you have the more your self-esteem and confidence goes up.

Cleanse your environment

The brain has deep wired connections between you and your environment. Are there places that you go to where they bring back deep seated memories that trigger happy or sad feelings?

Is so, your brain is reliving the experience and your hormones will react the same as the very first time, triggering cortisol for those upsetting memories. It is like reliving the event over and over again.

E.g. Break ups can be painful. You hold a lot of memories about your partner and your time together. It doesn't serve to dwell and relive the past. If you have energy around these triggers, it's time to sit with it and let it go.

Action: Spend time in each room of your house and think about how you feel when you are in that room, what feelings does it trigger? Do you feel calm and at peace or do you feel irritable? If you feel sad how can you change that? How can you make each room somewhere you love being?

Be authentic, be you

Don't be scared of being you. Don't be scared of showing your emotions. As hard as it may be, being vulnerable is one of your greatest strengths. Allow yourself to fully feel your fears and threats. If you have the courage to work with them and share them they become less scary to you.

Feeling fear is completely normal, but you mustn't allow it to define who you are. Without experiencing darkness you cannot truly know light. See a dichotomy, a contrast. Allow your light to shine bright.

When you are showing your true emotion and vulnerability others round you will feel empathy and connect with you. They will have the courage to do the same. It is part of being human, sharing real emotion isn't weak. Don't be ashamed or scared of it.

Action: Think about who or what has triggered your fear and what small steps you can take to make that fear less scary. If you are struggling with this find someone to talk to. It could be a friend, or a professional. Emotions always find a way out, even manifesting into physical pain or disease. They are form of energy and energy is meant to flow, energy in motion... e-motion. It's not about reliving painful memories, but allowing yourself to express them and fully feel them.

We are all unique, in fact we are unique EVERY single day. Yet we also human beings, and as humans our brains are wired in a certain way. Learn to understand how your brain works for you. Learn to forgive yourself and be kind to yourself often. Remember it is not in your mind, mind set or you it is how your brain was designed to work to keep you alive. By recognising this and accepting it allows you to move forwards. Having awareness when stressful triggers arise allows you to pause, breathe and respond differently instead of reacting and doing what you always do. Listen to what your body is telling you.

| 31 |

Self-Protection Starts With the Self

I abhor bullies.

I have done ever since I was at school. I kept out of trouble mostly, although I had a few skirmishes. But of those I did have I didn't like the horrific feeling surrounding it... FEAR.

So I embarked on my martial arts journey when I was 14, (now 35 years and counting), That's some journey.

I was inspired by Bruce lee, as most were back in the day. I wanted to punch and kick and just kick ass. Bruce was so cool. Before I even found a karate class I tried to emulate what he did. I seem to remember getting all of his films out from a video rental store, I could have only been 13, so I have no idea how I was able to rent them considering they were rated 18!

All those films did was fuel my fire more. I knew I had to find out more.

Then I remember watching the original Karate Kid back in 1984. I loved that movie and so found a book and tried to learn myself.

It wasn't until I was 15 that I found a class that looked great. The style was called Jintian Do, a mix of Tukido and Taekwondo and I loved it. I went with two friends, but they didn't last long, but I was hooked and never looked back.

I wanted to be a black belt to help protect myself.

Only when I got the coveted belt back when I was 17, nothing changed... at all. Yes I could fight, but that feeling never went away that feeling of being rooted to the spot, weak and terrified.

I had a run in with a local bully around that time and you know what? I was shit scared and ran away (well I locked myself in my car) until he left. I went home and I went through all the emotions...

Anger

Frustration

Embarrassment

Guilt

Shame

I didn't get it at the time. But I knew I couldn't live with these shit feelings and so I decided to go the bully's house to confront him.

I was still shit scared but I was NOT having this hanging over me. I knocked on the door and out he came. I challenged him there and then.

It turned out he was all bark and no bite, although he did bring his dog out to protect himself. He hid behind the dog with a volley of abuse and what he was going to do to me. I stood my ground and told him to put his dog away so I could settle this. He declined and retreated and I never saw him again.

So what has this got to do with you?

I will tell you.

FEAR.

Everyone goes through this every day; in their business, their relationships with their partners, kids, friends. I know I have. The feeling of not being good enough, not worthy enough, being judged.

All brought from FEAR.

Back then I was a good martial artist, I was fit and in good health (I still am) but back then I had felt paralysed by fear.

A few years later I sought out one of the world authorities in self-protection Geoff Thompson, to understand and get past fear of physical confrontations; to understand fear and all its guises. I travelled 500 miles every month for 5 years for his guidance and instruction... and brutal training sessions, man they were hard, not only physically, but mentally and emotionally. Every session challenged every fibre of my being. Every month I travelled to the classes, I had the urge to turn around and go home. But there is no growth in comfort.

Through the physical sessions and the metaphysical I came to realise I was here for so much more, I had an awakening that could not be reversed. I saw my true potential. Going through a forge tempers the blade, forcing myself to confront my thoughts and feelings. I saw that everything was waiting for me beyond my self-limiting beliefs, by leaning into my fears.

What I learned was priceless and I thought I would share it with you as it applies to anything in your life that you are afraid of confronting.

Self-protection starts with the self.

The physical stuff is the easy part. It's the inner bully that you have to master.

The ego.

The shadow.

The very thing preventing you from moving forwards and creating success in your career or business and living your dream life.

To stand up and defend yourself against YOUR inner bully takes courage... facing your adversity.

But to defend it, you have to know who you really are.

To strip down your very being, to lay it bare. To cut loose all the bull shit stories and old scripts and find your essence. Who you REALLY are.

No bravado or bull shit. The real person, most usually hiding away in a dark corner, afraid to show up in the world and step into the light.

Self-protection is self-sovereignty over the self. Supreme power of body, mind and spirit and it takes work, dedication, understanding and courage.

The thing is most people are absolutely terrified by their own potential. I was, in fact I still feel fear every day, but I know it is the path I get to walk to have what I want.

"Within my reach, but beyond my grasp."

I could see everything that was possible, but every time I moved towards it, I hit my invisible ceiling, my limiting beliefs, the old scripts and social mores rose up and I felt tremendous fear.

I know it can be debilitating. I have felt it myself in my business, but ignoring it and coming up with ways to ignore it and shy away, pretending it's not there or not what you want will never help you. You cannot hide from the person in the depths of your soul, screaming to get out...

Your purpose, your super power, the real reason you are on this spinning globe.

I would hear, "Who do you think you are? You are not good enough".

But understand this. They are just old scripts, automatically playing without challenge.

So challenge them!

You get to destroy old realities and create new ones simply by choosing to do so, any time you decide to.

Change is the only constant, but everyone is afraid of it.

There is almost always massive resistance, an urge to flee, your ego protecting you from yourself. That ego having been programmed by you to stay away from anything that feels unsafe. And change feels unsafe.

Most people do not know who they are. It's hard to articulate. But it is much easier to find out who you aren't and then what you stand for.

Find your essence, face your adversity.

Removing every single thing that does not serve you, stripping away the thoughts, possessions and people who drain you or distract you from your inner most fears. Then becoming a warrior, having the courage to face yourself.

So stand up to your inner bully. Recognise it is simply a reflection of your perception, your fears.

Challenge your perception, identify the person in the mirror.

Ask yourself are you happy?

And wait for your reply.

| 32 |

Where is Your Attention?

The only thing you truly need to work on is your attention. When I actually looked at this, I marvelled at its simplicity and power and then laughed at myself for being unaware of this simple truth.

Where are you placing your attention?

What you give your attention to, grows, what you take your attention away from, atrophies. Have you noticed? Our attention is scattered all the time. Your external world vies for your attention continuously, it is relentless!

I realised that most people cannot hold or control their attention. They often aren't even aware their attention is being taken away from them and so have no tools to take it back. The opportunity to respond differently starts with awareness.

How often have you found it impossible to focus your attention? I know it's been a constant struggle for me and I practise holding my attention every day. The more I practise this cerebral exercise, the stronger my attention becomes.

As with anything, it takes time and effort with more than a hint of discipline to control your attention. After all, what we place our attention on, we bring life to.

This is why so many people struggle with meditation. Meditation requires you to place your attention on one thing; a chime, a sound, a mantra or breathing. Holding your focus in one spot takes discipline as your attention wants to scatter in all directions. Your thoughts lead you all over the place. Practising focussing your attention in meditation allows you to recognise when your mind drifts, so you can refocus.

Your reality is created from where you place your attention every day. Stop and think about that for a minute. If your focus is locked into fear, scarcity and lack, you will attract more of the same.

And yet fear is so prevalent. It is fed to you in the newspapers and on the news every minute of every day. Misery and sensationalism sells and makes money for the media; they are not interested in you or your health remember that.

Consider the main stories; wars, abuse, killing, affairs, gossip, soaps, celebrity; all excessive information that feeds your fears. They take your attention to dark places.

If you feed on these stories, take them in and believe them, that becomes who you are. Your attention becomes locked on survival. Will I have money? Am I safe to walk the streets? Is it safe to go abroad? All fear based thoughts; all driving you to live from a place of fear. No wonder there is so much depression and anxiety in the world, so much energy draining away unnecessarily.

Because people haven't got control of their attention, they are not even aware that they are giving it away every time they are distracted listening to stories that do not serve them at all.

But what if you stopped? What if you put attention onto your thoughts or what you were about to say; asking yourself 'is this useful?' What if you found better information; inspiring and empowering information that lifts you up instead of bringing you down?

So where is your attention right now? If it's not where you want it to be, then you have the power to course correct.

Where do you want to place you attention?

Mine is on self-development, curiosity and wonder of what's possible; mastery of the physical body, optimising my physical, mental, emotional and spiritual well-being. What I can achieve, how I want to live. I get my information from inspiring sources; books, people. I am interested in finding the essence of me, who I am stripped back and then changing my reality by removing who I am not and creating space for a reality that inspires me.

I don't need a newspaper to tell me a skewed view of what is going on in the world. I have my own 'sat nav'. You have it too; it's called intuition. If I create space to listen, it guides me to better more exciting information so I can let go of old perceptions to create new ones that serve me.

Ultimately we do not want to be surviving, stuck in fear sponsored thoughts and feelings. We want to be thriving, to be free, fulfilled and have an abundant life. The ability to choose where you place (and don't place) your attention is true freedom.

But so many people are not free. If they are insulted in some way it takes away their attention, their energy is placed in the insult that can last for days. The opposite is also true, being praised lifts their spirits but their attention is still taken away; being at the mercy of someone else's comments, opinions and energy both good and bad.

Their attention being determined by external influences, what they think, what they were told, what they read, instead of being in control they are being controlled.

When I train in the martial arts, my attention is absolute. My focus is on awareness of my opponent, looking to score my own hits whilst not being punched or kicked or choked out. It is being in my centre, controlling the uncomfortable feelings of which there are many and being disciplined. That environment demands your attention.

The same applies to addictive behaviours. Those behaviours steal your attention. If you step back and observe the thoughts and feelings around those behaviours and not engage, you can take your attention back.

It could be the urge to overeat that comes up and you cannot hold your attention in a healthy place. Attention is stolen by the need to have excess and you lose control of your attention. So, instead of automatically reaching for food, stop, breath and observe where your attention is going, and what it brings up for you.

Having the ability to hold your attention allows for self-mastery, being in control of your body and mind. Have the discipline to recognise the thoughts and sensations and not engage or be distracted; simply detach and observe what is going on in your body.

Yes I know it's not easy, but it is possible. It takes work, practice and dedication. But I ask you, who wouldn't want to be in control of their attention in today's fast paced world?

Think about the big stealers of your attention right now, phones, texts, social media all vying to steal your time and energy away. Does that really serve you? Is that what you really want?

You can make up reasons and excuses, but you always know deep down. It's having the courage to admit it to yourself and bring your attention to what is really going on.

You can soon find out if you are in control. Try and stop something that takes your attention. If you are unable to, you are not in control, someone or something else is. Think about that for a minute.

We can practise attention every day; locking your attention into something right in front of you, complete focus on the task at hand.

Do you give your full attention to your children or your partner, are you being present in the moment, or are you on your phone or watching TV or thinking about work?

You can change this by choosing to respond differently. If you have the urge to overeat, stop and calm your mind through focussed breathing. Resist the urge to react and identify the driving thought. Feel the sensation. What triggered it? Allow yourself to feel that trigger until it dissipates.

Controlling the palate is the best way to control your attention. It brings awareness to the thoughts and associations around not only food but whatever you take in via your senses.

How do you start? With the breath. Keep bringing awareness to your environment, what you are thinking, saying and doing; bring awareness to how it is affecting you. What are you allowing to take your attention away from you? What are you allowing to take control of you?

You can choose where to put your attention at any moment. You can create the reality in your life that you want to create by bringing awareness to your attention.

| 33 |

Brain Training

I have seen so many people as titans in areas of physical fitness. They look after their physical body with all manner of activities and sport, which is great. However, as you are in no doubt aware by now, this is only one element of health I believe in, just one piece of the jigsaw. I also see so many of the same people who are minnows in the mental arena, who as fit as they are physically are not doing the work mentally.

Very quickly in the realms of what I believe health is, you realise that it's not if a person can get better, it's whether their belief systems let them and whether they are open to exploring and dispelling beliefs that hold them back. Beliefs form part of your identity and if you are not open and brave enough to challenge those beliefs, you will remain stuck.

This is why so many people experience pain. Installed beliefs can create anxiety and stress, which overstimulates the nervous system. That heightened fear and worry can create more protection than is needed (remember, 'Am I safe?').

Brain training or mental fitness is just as important as physical fitness, and yet most people do not do it. They focus on their physical fitness, but neglect the grey matter between their ears.

Focusing on the foundation of health will keep the brain in tip top condition to find that peak state where we can use our brain for all manner of tasks and create amazing things.

The mind is a muscle and we get to flex and train it. Through neuroscience we now know about neuro plasticity, the ability to change and rewire the brain, removing neural connections that are no longer necessary or useful and strengthening others to become even more mentally strong, healthy and fit.

Mental fitness means optimising your mental and emotional health. Making make sure you are looking after your brain, giving it the nutrients it needs and being in the human part of your brain more often.

Making sure you have mental and emotional resilience is important. Being in control of your thoughts and feelings allows for increased confidence and clarity of mind and building self-acceptance, self-esteem and having the courage to be you.

By making sure your foundational needs are met more often, you can access the creative, human part of your brain, the neocortex, allowing you to think critically, creatively and logically.

Sometimes it is not so much about adding than subtracting. It's about letting go of what thoughts that do not serve you so you can make room for those that do. It's important to realise that you are not your thoughts. You do not have to engage in thoughts that do not serve you. Practising the art of bringing awareness to your thoughts and observing them without reacting to them is essential for your mental fitness.

Where to Start?

Creating a good foundation. Using the basic principles of variety and curiosity think about what can challenge you. Think of skills to learn that you have never tried, get curious about the world and how things work.

Expand your mind and look at what is truly possible. Daydream, use your powerful imagination, read far and wide. Look at the religious texts, the philosophers and the unsung heroes. Find inspiration from those who have triumphed over adversity. Find humour in your life, smile, laugh and laugh some more. There is not one single rule that life has to be taken so seriously.

Give yourself time each day to slow down and decompress. Make it a priority to contemplate and reflect and let go of things that do not serve you.

Physical activity helps your mind as well as your body. Physical activity increases the flow of oxygen to your brain, increasing the level of 'feel good' endorphins in your brain. It's no surprise that people with good physical fitness have better mental agility. Physical activity can alleviate anxiety and depression and help create a more positive outlook on life.

Meditation is a great way of calming the mind and bringing you back to your centre. It allows you to practise controlled breathing and awareness of your thoughts, practising keeping your attention and defending yourself against your 'inner bully'.

Challenge your intellect and memory. Stretch yourself mentally by learning a new language, doing the cryptic crossword, learning a new language or playing chess. There are now brain training apps that challenge your memory, visualisation and reasoning. Find something that challenges your mental capacity often. This is important for brain health and good for your social life.

Learning something new gives the 'grey matter' a workout and builds neural pathways in the brain. It could be anything like something physical that involves coordination such as a martial art, skipping, dancing or juggling or learning a new skill such as woodwork, model building, playing a musical instrument or drawing and painting. Something that you enjoy that is a challenge.

Nutrition also optimises your mental fitness, optimising your gut health which is directly connected to your brain and is known as the 2nd brain and controlling your blood sugars will lower brain inflammation.

Adding Omega 3 fish oils are essential for brain health. Either supplement or eat oily fish 3-4 times per week (salmon, sardines, mackerel, herring etc).

Eat more antioxidants. These protect from oxidative stress that protects the brain. Berries are a great source, packed full of protective compounds.

Vitamin B from things like salmon, sardines, beef or tuna and folate from green leafy vegetables is also essential for good brain health.

Hydration is hugely important. Around 75% of brain weight is water. Mental performance is affected when we are dehydrated and it doesn't take much to be hydrated. Ask yourself how often do you replace lost fluids.

Sleep, rest and recovery are essential and help reduce the other thing that can have a big detrimental effect on the brain... stress.

PART V – SPIRITUAL HEALTH

| 34 |

Who is the Real Me?

Spirituality is the fourth piece of the health jigsaw. I have seen the word spirituality often confused with religion. I mixed up the two for the longest time.

Spirituality and religion are not the same thing, although they kind of overlap. They share similarities such as belief, comfort, reflection and contemplation.

I see spirituality as a sense of connection to something bigger than ourselves. We are all children of this world. We are all connected, energetic beings after all. It may just not feel like it right now.

Ask yourself why that is?

The problem we face is that we live in a materialistic, commercial world, with the majority of people too busy focused on the next 'thing' thinking it will make them happy. But happiness is a state of being, a choice we get to make remember? It's not in the next purchase we make.

There is a lack of awareness in most people because there are so many external distractions and that is easier to focus on rather than doing the internal work. Why? Because starting to go within feels scary. It's easier to be distracted, trying to fit in with everyone else rather than listening to what your heart tells you, trusting in who you are and standing out.

But what if 'fitting in' is not the answer and has never been?

Spiritual health can mean different things to different people, however I believe it is reconnecting to your soul, expressing what sets your soul on fire, that burning desire that is not influenced by external things. The place where you feel most at home, at peace, finding the meaning and purpose of your life, living by your values and what you stand for and against.

"If you really want to be brave, if you really want peace, then stop going out and start going within."

– DEAN COULSON

Very few do this kind of soul searching and yet taking the courage to just stop and listen to your heart can be so liberating.

Spirituality is state of being, not a state of doing. It is letting go of the meanings and emotions we attach to things. Having the ability to stay calm amongst the chaos, sitting in that eye wall of a storm and letting go of the drama.

Drama being events and situations that we give a certain meaning to. The emotional connection we attach to them that allows us to create that chaos. It's easy to blame other people or things for how we feel and yet no one can make us feel anything, we allow it to happen.

Being able to master your own mental and emotional state and not being attached to external influences or meanings is powerful and is part of self-mastery. Having that sense of calm and inner peace, away from fear and uncertainty.

Having a clear definition of we you are and who we choose to be and letting go of things that do not align with that.

We all carry emotional baggage, anchors from our past that pull us out of balance. It's learning to let go of these emotions and forgiving ourselves. You can feel when energy around you is up or down, even if you cannot quite explain it or even believe it.

I feel spiritual health goes beyond a sensory experience, it's about letting go of the attachments to time, body and the environment, (no time, no-body, no place). Letting go of the influences that we allow to control us, the things that we allow to create our identity and how we exist in this world.

I love the idea of purging, finding your essence and letting go of all the things that do not serve you. It can be a daunting task; you attach meaning to situations and circumstances, objects and possessions. Understanding why you have labelled them as important will recoup that energy for more purposeful things. It is the art of reduction, finding out who you are by knowing who you are not then letting it go, trusting your intuition and having the faith it will be ok.

Ask yourself what you have in your life and whether it serves a purpose. If it doesn't why do you have it? What are you clinging on to? Why is it important to you?

The things anchored in our past, defining who we are, are not set in stone. Spiritual health is letting go of those connections, being in the moment, almost like obsessing about a new positive, desired experience that you haven't yet embraced emotionally.

Realising that all we ever need we already have.

It's never about have – do – be, but be – do – have.

Ask yourself who you would love to be. Imagine what that would be like. How would you think, act and feel. Ask yourself what that person would do in this moment and be thankful as if it had already happened, giving it over to the universe, that higher energetic force.

It's not about cause and effect. It's about causing an effect. Being that person now and influencing who you are right now. You don't require something to happen first. Happiness is a choice, you get to be that right now if you let go of that expectation, those mind forged manacles keeping you stuck.

Be aware of what energy you are sending out, the frequency you are operating from. If that is fear, scarcity and lack, guess what will come back to you? More of the same. When you find yourself in a fearful situation, ask yourself, "What would love do?"

Reconnect With Yourself

It can feel scary to explore new realities for ourselves as we have attached beliefs and stories to our identities and it can feel unsafe if we try and let go. The ego will fight tooth and nail to hold on.

However, if you understand that the ego only exists in time, where it anchors itself in the past to dictate your future using your experiences, stories and beliefs to steer you, you can then take back control.

The thing is, the ego is a good servant but a bad master. You get to take control of that, by surrendering and letting go of the anchors of the past and keeping your mind in the present, you are lightening the load.

By letting go of the people, possessions and circumstances that drain you and focus on surrounding yourself with inspiring people you can change your environment in line with who you deeply desire to be.

Protect your energy at all costs. Your energy is finite, everything you think say and do takes your energy. It's amazing how much we give away and the attachments we cling on to.

Ask yourself, "How much energy am I giving away so needlessly? How can I take that back? What do I need to do to take my power back?"

Take steps to halt the energy drain. Who is draining you? What is draining you? What can you stop doing today that serves no purpose?

It's time to slow down your world, empty your cup, let go of the superfluous, whatever does not serve you. Be brutally honest with yourself. Step back and take a 30000 feet view and really look at is what is going on in your life. Make it a daily ritual to slow down, stop and bring awareness through your senses. What is going on right now? Not what you are projecting into your future based on experiences from your past.

Look at doing something that uplifts you to reconnect with yourself and your higher purpose. That could be volunteering work or working with a charity. It might be expressing yourself, reconnecting with your heart, writing poetry, writing song lyrics, dancing, singing, walking in nature. Everyone has a natural bias, what is yours? How can you create more fulfilment?

| 35 |

Do you Mind?

Since humans spend so much time being out of their minds, 3 brains remember? It's important to create space to stop. In fact it's important to give yourself permission to prioritise some time for your wellbeing. So many people tell me they don't have the time. Well I simply don't agree.

It is those same people who spend too long in front of a TV or mindlessly scrolling through social media.

I invite you to consider that it's never about the lack of time, it is more about setting incorrect priorities. Every person on this planet has access to the same amount of time, it is always about how you choose to spend it.

Where some people move mountains and create successful, fulfilled lives, others squander their time and blame this shortage of time on anything and everything but the life they lead.

I know I have been there and it sucks. I have squandered time and apportioned blame. But who does that really serve? It didn't serve me at all. It was just an energy drain. When your brain doesn't feel safe you will spin your wheels and get nowhere. It comes back to listening to your heart, allowing yourself to fully feel those 'unsafe' feelings and recognise the habitual patterns.

Allow yourself to pause, stop and create space to just be. You don't have to be busy all of the time. That is most often a distraction to stop you feeling what your brain has labelled as unsafe. If you want to stop going round in circles in your life create space to slow down and stop; prioritising time for yourself is a top priority. Your time and energy is a finite resource and you get to protect it at all costs.

Mindfulness

Mindfulness is the art of being in the moment, being consciously aware of your surroundings, the sights and sounds, the smells and sensations. It is the ability to have complete presence and teaching you awareness of what is happening in your body and mind and being open to it with curiosity and kindness.

It allows you to explore your own beliefs, perspectives and experiences in a different light, leading to new questions and answers.

Because mindfulness is the practice of awareness in the present moment it can help if you struggle with things such as overeating or persistent snacking, feeling anxious or depressed, feeling distracted or struggle with your concentration, stress or even being kind to yourself.

It takes practise; you may find your mind wandering, but just like any kind of training, the longer you do it, the easier it becomes until it becomes second nature. Nothing worth doing is easy. It takes commitment to being consistent every day, even when you don't feel like it. Make it non-negotiable.

Simple ways to practice mindfulness:

Living in the moment. Being present, aware of what is happening right in front of you. Finding joy in the simplest of pleasures, having an immersive conversation or eating a meal, experiencing the taste and textures and how your body reacts to the food.

Paying attention. Taking notice of everything around you. How you feel, observing your thoughts, Using your senses and tuning in to the sights and sounds around you. Slowing down and enjoying the experience.

Self-acceptance. Being kind to yourself. Treating yourself as you would your best friend.

Breathing. The most powerful tool in your mindfulness toolbox. The ability to breathe diaphragmatically (See the 'Take a Deep Breath' chapter for more details) and take back control. Focus on the breath, slow it down, breathe out at least as slow as breathing in. You can do this anywhere.

Sitting with your feelings. Allowing yourself to fully feel whatever you are experiencing. Notice where you are experiencing sensations in the body and focus on them until they fade away.

Remember, mindfulness isn't a something thing, it's an all-time thing. Create the space in your day to practise.

| 36 |

What Are You Grateful For?

It's funny how we can go through life just taking things for granted. I certainly have. There are times when I have had no awareness of how everyone and everything I have in my life are so amazing. And I have certainly seen the outcome of that ignorance...

Anxiety, stress, overwhelm, frustration, anger.

Gratitude goes way beyond please and thank you. I see more and more when I don't practise gratitude, when I fall out of alignment of who I am, I find myself focusing on the wrong things...

Why has my business idea not worked?

Why are they having a go at me?

Why did that client not ring me back?

Why is this process so difficult?

Why is someone being ungrateful?

What have I done to deserve this?

It's not my fault!

When this happens I realise one thing. I am not practising gratitude myself.

The HUGE red flag.

So I remind myself that all of those thoughts don't matter and I focus on the things I am grateful for, what IS important to me. I can only see in others what I see in myself. So if I find myself criticising or judging, that is all on me. Otherwise, I just wouldn't see it, there would be no resonance. That tells me that I am not taking time to do the work.

That's when I work on my inner game. Understanding that anything that triggers me, every reaction I have to something I don't like or more often what reminds me of something painful, even if that is unconscious, has nothing to do with anyone but me. If my thoughts, words and deeds are not happy, kind and courteous, then I have something inside to address.

I get to choose whether to understand and improve myself or ignore it and stay in the pity party (and I have hosted plenty of those!). We get so focused chasing things we don't have, that we forget to be GRATEFUL for what we DO have. We get caught up in what we are not getting, we forget the wonderful things right in front of us.

When was the last time you STOPPED thinking about all the things you want to achieve or what you haven't got and think about what you already have?

I check in with my health constantly. I challenge thoughts I have, the words I say and the actions I take and whether that compromises me in any way. It is so easy to take health for granted. It is a gift that is so often abused. I know I have. But now if shit shows up to compromise that? I challenge it.

If you are in good health, you have all your limbs, you can see, hear, smell and taste, if you can walk and exercise, be grateful.

If you have a family, wife, kids, parents, friends. Be grateful.

These are things to be grateful for, which the majority of us take for granted. I know I have, too often. Don't wait until you haven't got these things to realise what you had was so precious.

Be grateful today.

I was recently asked what was one thing I was grateful for, my answer? Breathing. Every morning when I open my eyes I give thanks that I have another day on this planet to experience life regardless of how I am feeling. Placing my thoughts in a place of gratitude allows me to set my mind to higher frequency where I can operate from a place of love.

Practise gratitude now and every day. Stop and think about what wonderful things you have and really appreciate that you have them. Focus on the abundance all around you and not the things you lack. One comes from a place of love, the other from fear. It is so easy to place your whole focus on one small thing that isn't going right and forget about all the other things we have that are really more important, what is going right? What is amazing?

So what is really important to you that you may be taking for granted?

If it's your health, take steps to improve it.

If it is a relationship with yourself, your partner, your siblings, your parents, friends, then be thankful to yourself and those you hold dear.

If it is your job or business; how can you help more people get what they want?

Gratitude opens the door and closes the door

It opens the gate and closes the gate.

Gratitude is the way to an abundant life you choose.

How grateful are you for the life you lead?

| 37 |

Forgive Yourself

It is important to recognise that we are not perfect, in fact perfection doesn't exist. All we can do is to strive to be all that we are, by letting go of who we are not. There will be a time when we make mistakes. The thing is, it's ok to err, its ok to lose our way.

From my own experience and study, everyone makes mistakes, I know I have. It is whether we can admit to them and forgive our mistakes and move on without allowing them to define who we are.

We are often at our most harsh when we make mistakes. It's one thing forgiving others but much harder forgiving yourself. I have been there, in fact I am still working on it, every day.

I would forgive my son

I would forgive my wife

I would forgive my family

I would forgive my friend

But then I would beat myself up and be so hard on myself and for what?

To make myself feel shit. How does that serve me?

Being so self-critical and self-judgemental certainly didn't help me; it didn't make me feel good at all.

When we make mistakes we can feel anger, shame and guilt; All low vibrating energies. We fear the judgement it may bring. I have been in that place of berating myself and calling myself names. In reality though, that is simply an expectation set by ourselves or someone else that we are not meeting. It is all part of the human experience.

That's when I took a different perspective. To conserve my energy and let things go. To accept that some days 'it' just beats you.

Sometimes the anger beats you

Sometimes the frustration beats you

Sometimes the judgement beats you

Sometimes the jealousy beats you

Sometimes the envy beats you

Sometimes it just beats you. Whatever it is... And that's ok.

It means you are on the right path and there are lessons to learn, feelings to experience and thoughts to contemplate. If you don't have days when you feel beaten, you are not in the right place. You are not challenging yourself enough to grow, to feel discomfort. You are not asking the right questions of yourself.

Of course we don't want to keep making mistakes, but if we continue to strive and challenge ourselves, being in discomfort, they will appear. Those mistakes or failures are simply lessons to show us where to go next. We are not perfect, but we do not need to be. If we cannot forgive ourselves then we are not living in the present moment, we are allowing our past to dictate our future.

Don't be so hard on yourself.

Allow yourself to feel that energy you are feeling and let it go. Let go of the guilt and shame, let go of the anger and frustration. Ask yourself "What am I really angry about?" Learn from the mistakes and move forward.

Breathe, give yourself a break and take it easy on yourself.

Everything will be ok, I promise.

| 38 |

Kill Them with Kindness

Are you kind to yourself? I don't just mean sometimes, I mean all of the time? Do you listen to the language you use with yourself, especially when you are alone? Your thoughts and words count. They make an impact and if you are not being kind to yourself with every internal interaction then it will impact your mental health and emotional wellbeing.

Being kind is about giving without thought of reward, being generous with your time and energy just because you can. Simply allowing your heart to open and being kind in your thoughts, words and actions.

Kindness starts with you. Always remember to prioritise time for you every day. It may sound trivial but how often do you bring awareness to your internal dialog?

Are you being unkind to yourself?

Are you being unkind to others?

Nothing good comes from hate or vitriol. It takes the same energy to be kind as it is to be mean. If we are projecting hate and anger ask yourself what is really going on? What is driving it?

If you are calling yourself names, ask if that is really justified? If you are getting involved in gossip does it actually serve you? Do you actually believe it or are you joining in to fit in? Is it being kind?

It takes no effort to be kind; offering a word of encouragement, a smile or a thank you. Being kind is a way to connect with others in a deep and meaningful way.

Have compassion by understanding that we don't know how other people feel, how other people's lives are. Anger and frustrations come from some expectation that isn't being met. If that anger is directed towards you, it isn't about you. You have just become a mirror, showing them a reflection they do not like. A reminder of what they haven't done or are unwilling to do.

They are not attacking you; they are reacting to being reminded of something they do not like. That's all on them, you do not have to defend yourself or prove them wrong for you to be right, just have compassion for what they might be going through in their lives.

Look at your day right now, have you been kind to yourself?

Was every thought kind?

Was every word kind?

Was every action kind?

To you and to those around you?

It takes massive introspection to challenge the stories we believe to allow kindness to shine through. Bringing awareness to every thought, word and action from a place of love and compassion allows you to thrive in your life.

Make your kindness intentional, perform voluntary acts of kindness. What can you do today to be kind?

Here are a few thoughts… Volunteer to help, give compliments, donate to a charity, hold a door, let someone have your seat, offer your expertise to those who are struggling, check in with your neighbours, help in your community, call a friend, litter pick, buy a stranger a coffee. I'm sure you can come up with more.

Kindness makes you feel good, it keeps things in perspective and it keeps you in alignment to your values.

THINK!

Too many people open their mouths without thinking. Ask yourself whether what you are saying...

T - Is it even true, have you challenged it?

H - Is it helpful to you or others?

I - Is it inspiring, does it set your soul on fire?

N - Is it necessary, is it useful?

K - Is it kind or is it hurtful?

Make a positive impact by choosing what you say to yourself and others wisely. Be kind!

| 39 |

Meditation

One way to optimise and practise spiritual health and wellbeing is through meditation.

With the hectic pace and demands of modern life, many people feel stressed and over-worked every day. Our stress and tiredness make us unhappy, impatient and frustrated as we don't give ourselves time to slow down. Meditation is one of the most overlooked forms of training and yet mastering it can yield amazing health benefits by creating an inner space and clarity that enables us to control our mind regardless of the external circumstances.

Meditation opens the gate to who we are, bypassing our conscious filters (how we view the world) so we can access our unconscious mind and move away from being our thoughts and beliefs to observing them, and changing them to be more productive.

Meditation allows you to reassert control over the subconscious programmes that have run you for too long. You get to stop being the old you, to make room for a new personality. Finding your connection to your source, that meaning and purpose, why you are here on this spinning orb. What allows you access to your inner self? Connecting to something bigger than you.

The reason people shy aware from mediation, why they say they are too busy or it doesn't work, its stupid etc is really none of those things. It is being alone with their thoughts. In fact when I started meditating all manner of distracting thoughts came into my head to prevent me from doing it.

In fact that still happens, but I just smile as I am aware of the minds tricks. Whatever the mind thinks is unapproachable or is unsafe it will try to distract with whatever has worked before to keep you safe.

But how does that serve you?

Silence is deafening, it unsettles us because once we shut out the external world through meditation, our thoughts seem to amplify and that can feel overwhelming. Remember, we are not our thoughts. We can bring awareness to them and observe them or engage with them.

The idea is not to clear your mind of thoughts, considering we have as many as 6000 thoughts every day. It's allowing the flow of your thoughts without engagement. Just as with physical health, getting in the gym and lifting the weights strengthens muscles.

Meditation is like a mind gym, doing the reps and sets to train the mind. Observing but not engaging your thoughts, practising awareness when you do engage a thought to then bring your mind back to your centre.

Just like any workout, whether it is physical or mental it is challenging but ultimately worthwhile. The more you do it the more control you will have. Meditation is a tool to allow the mind total freedom to explore and let go of any expectation.

I remember being frustrated when I started meditating simply because I had placed an expectation on what I was doing; like I would reach some spiritual nirvana. In reality I realised I was frightened of what it might show me. Meditation takes time and practise. It is not a quick fix, it takes a lifetime of dedication to master your mind but why wouldn't you want to have that control?

When it comes to meditation there tends to be a habit of interchanging mindfulness and awareness, but I believe they are different.

Mindfulness brings focus to what you are doing and your surroundings in the present moment, being conscious of what you think, say and do, for example, brushing your teeth, eating or washing your hands. Focusing on the task at hand.

The practice of awareness is more about focusing on one thing, whether it is your breathe or a single sound, for example in practising meditation.

Meditation, changes the relationship you have with your thoughts and emotions, it's not about getting rid of them. It's a way to connect to the essence of who you are.

As much as there are guided meditations, I don't believe that is really meditation, it is engaging thoughts through prompts and you can become reliant on some external voice. By meditating in silence or focus on a single object allows the mind freedom to explore without any reliance on a prompt.

Meditation reduces stress and allows you to gain a greater mastery over thoughts and emotions, but also to discover your minds deep potential for unconditional compassion and freedom to allow your happiness to shine.

How to Meditate

There are a myriad of books on mediation, I wanted to share with you a simple way to get started. You can either sit in a comfortable upright position or lie down in a quiet place. I will be honest I prefer sitting to lying down, When I lie down my body knows it's time to sleep and shuts down. Find your own position that feels safe to you.

If you haven't tried to meditate before, start with 5-10 minutes and work up from there until you can do 20-30 mins. Control your breathing pattern by focusing on the breath. Breathe diaphragmatically by inhaling through the nose for 4 seconds, pause and exhaling for 4 seconds, pause again and repeat. If your mind starts to wander bring your attention back to the breath.

The best time to meditate is in the morning. We tend to wake up with a mind full of chaos and 'things to do'; meditation allows you to create space, slow things down and bring you back to your centre. Our stress hormone cortisol is part of our circadian rhythm, the sleep/wake cycle and rises naturally to wake you up in the morning. Meditating at this time can level cortisol off and bring a calmness and focus to the start of your day.

PART VI – TIME TO THRIVE!

| 40 |

Reconstructing Yourself

Since you ultimately shaped your world and created your current reality through your past conditioning and experiences, you have the ability to destroy that reality and create a new one any time you choose.

Easier said than done I hear you say!

And I agree with you.

Nothing worth doing is ever easy.

Self-development is one of the toughest challenges you will ever face. Very few step into the arena of the internal game. It is uncomfortable; it is painful and is unrelenting. But that is why you are here right, because you want more from your life? You want to understand who you are, know what you stand for and be strong in your truth; to develop resilience in each realm... physical, mental, emotional and spiritual. You want to thrive and that takes total commitment.

Commitment – a promise, declaration or decision that you do not relent on no matter what circumstances arise; a choice that will liberate you from your fears.

Self-development is incredibly rewarding. It takes courage to be vulnerable, to say, "Here I am warts and all. This is me and I'm ok with that." I see vulnerability as having the courage to do something without any control of the outcome. Many think vulnerability is a weakness but I believe it is your greatest strength. Courage is not built in a vacuum, you have to step up and do something tangible in spite of how you feel.

The world is ripe with excuse makers not taking responsibility or owning up. Do you accept excuses into your world? If you are not moving forward and are apportioning blame, no matter how relevant it may be to you, that is still a barrier you are putting up to prevent your ascension. You take your power back by taking full responsibility. It's not about saving face, it's about stepping up and owning it.

If you have come this far then maybe you are willing to go a bit further; to put into practice what you have learned; to challenge the beliefs you have; to search out the truth; to trust your intuition; to challenge the narrative running in your head; to create daily rituals and impeccable agreements that you do not compromise on to keep taking the steps. Stay in the eye of the storm, your centre, when the shit hits the fan and everything around you descends into chaos.

The information in this book gives you the tools and resources to literally rebuild your life; to create daily practices; to construct a new path; to understand what health is, how you can optimise it and what can hold you back and how to resolve it.

To allow yourself to see that, you get to choose how your life will be and remove the obstacles you may not have even realised were even there. There will be resistance and you will question things and that is fine. You will know deep down whether the answers are a truth or a lie, IF you allow yourself to listen to what your heart tells you.

No one is coming to save you. You have to decide whether to play the blame game and stay in a victim state, or take responsibility for all your thoughts, words actions and be a victor. One makes your heart contract; the other makes your heart expand. You have a choice to make, whether to continue to talk about change or being the change in your actions.

Make no mistake. It takes time, energy and unrelenting effort. It is knowing when to step up and when to back off, trusting your intuition and not allowing your head to rule your heart.

Giving yourself permission to let go of the thoughts, words and actions that have held you captive for so long is liberating... and achievable.

| 41 |

Awareness, Avoidance, Escape

I have spent many years in the martial arts and have learned skills from some incredible people. One such person is Geoff Thompson, a world authority in self-protection who I sought out when I wanted to know about fear and how to better protect myself and my family from violent confrontations. His story resonated with me and so I embarked on a 5 year pilgrimage to Coventry, a 500 mile round trip every month to learn from the very best.

What I learned was way beyond what I ever could have imagined and not what I was expecting. It brought a new awareness to my life. The lessons were right in front of me hidden in plain sight waiting for me to see them. I began to see what is truly possible if I removed the blinkers of my conditioning and beliefs so I could see.

The foundation of physical self-protection is awareness, avoidance, escape and if all else fails pre-emption, striking first and striking hard (as long as you firmly believe you are in danger of serious harm) so as to escape. But why does this matter to you reading this book about thriving?

These foundations hold the same value against your inner bully, your inner opponent; the voice inside your head which always seems to stop you in your tracks when you want to change some or all of your life.

Self-protection always starts with the self. Defending against your inner bully (ego), the voice you hear in your head that stops you from moving forwards. This voice raises questions that can lead to self-doubt based on old cognitions that were placed there at some point in your past.

But why does it feel at times that your ego is against you?

You might even think the ego is your enemy but it is not. It simply acts on the stories and beliefs you have taken as your truth and they are then used to keep you safe; physically, mentally, emotionally and spiritually.

Past conditioning, society, old scripts and stories are used as a blueprint by the ego to form part of your identity. But that doesn't mean they are cast in stone. What you believe is transient and can be changed as long as you are aware, open minded and courageous enough to find a way to do so that the brain feels safe.

That starts with awareness; realising you can transform your life if you choose to do so. Awareness precedes change. Only you can challenge the dialog of your inner bully, you can challenge what is true for you. Only you can ask questions and feel the energetic return, which lets you know what to look at and what to let go of. When you stop engaging and start observing your thoughts and feelings you will be able to look objectively at what your ego is saying and respond differently. One thing to realise right now is you are NOT your thoughts.

In physical self-protection, people who are unaware or unprepared and oblivious to their environment and any threat that exists are known to be living in code white. This is a reference to the cooper colour codes relating to the level of threat in your environment, who is in it, where you are, how dangerous it is. This is when people are most vulnerable, showing a lack of awareness of their surroundings.

This applies to your inner bully too; having no awareness that the inner bully is calling the shots and not being in control of your thoughts and blindly following them without recourse. You are reacting to situations that have some emotional resonance without any control what will happen.

Just as in physical self-protection, awareness, avoidance, escape and pre-emption apply to our inner bully too. Let's delve further...

Awareness - of what you think, say, do and feel at any moment. Whether it is incongruent or out of alignment with your values. You get to bring awareness to what you are thinking and feeling. By having awareness you can respond in a manner that serves you. You feel stuck if you don't feel you are living life as the best version of yourself. The first step is realising that you can choose differently even if it feels hard or painful. You can either run away or face the consequences of your action or inaction. Challenge everything and make sure it is right for you.

Avoidance. Changing what does not serve you, let go of past beliefs and stories. Focusing on what you do want. To reiterate, your energy flows where your focus goes. Have the courage to let go of what no longer serves you, no matter what it is. Do not compromise on things that matter to you.

Escape – Sometimes you do not realise you are in a prison until you escape from it. You cannot see the picture when you are stuck inside the frame. The mind can keep you a prisoner of your own thoughts and beliefs. You have the opportunity to leave your addictive behaviours behind any time you choose, those repeating patterns that have kept you stuck; cutting ties with the addictions that have fed on you for so long. You may think that you have no addictions. You might be in denial that some thought or belief is keeping you prisoner. So let us consider what an addiction actually means. Addiction isn't about morals and ethics; addiction is about cause and effect. If the cause is excessive the effect is often addiction. So many people are locked in their own fears, justifying an existence. But who really wants to just exist? Once you escape you realise how much you were trapped.

Pre-emption - Live life proactively, with intention. Don't wait for permission how to live your life. Believe in yourself and why you were put on this planet. You do not have to prove anyone wrong for you to be right about you. You must be bold, brazen and unapologetically you. By stepping forward you are testing your perceived limits, proving to yourself that everything is ok. Taking a step out of faith that feels good to you, encourages you to take another to prove to yourself it can be done. Do not wait for someone else to say it's ok. You take the lead. Find others who have done what you want to do. Look for the evidence and blaze your own trail. Take aligned action, do the work.

| 42 |

Your Commitments

Have you ever considered your commitments to yourself?

Have you really thought about what you are doing and why you are doing it? I mean creating space to be alone without distraction or influence and asking why?

What actions are you taking with regards to your physical, mental, emotional and spiritual health? Do they align with what you said you wanted?

Have you ever considered that the commitments you have made in your life so far have led you to this point? If those commitments have led you to bliss in every part of your life then that is fantastic, but if they haven't, where are you falling short and how do you feel about it?

Does that sting? It did for me. I remember not being in a good place. My coach at that time revealed this truth to me and I reacted, not in a good way. I knew I wasn't living up to my own potential and I was out of alignment, but I didn't want to believe I had created a reality I did not like. I remember thinking it wasn't my fault!

It was circumstance, it was his fault, it was her fault, it was their fault, it was, it was... ME!

Damn, that hit hard. But when I just stopped and accepted that truth it was also so empowering. It meant I could change it. It was in my control. I could take back my power. I had to take responsibility for every single thing. I realised that I had been making excuses and avoiding certain situations and placing blame outside of me, when I knew it lay at my door. Some of it didn't make me feel good, but when it comes down to your emotional wellbeing, you get to express who you are. It is those feelings that lead you to your gold. You can try and avoid them but they will continue to come back round until you address them. Those sensations are what you get to face and fully feel and let go of. Acceptance is the first step to taking your power back.

You will always go out of your way to prove your unconscious beliefs true and you always get what you commit to. So if that is poor health, poor relationships (with yourself and others) or poor financial circumstances then this is a reflection of something deeper that has not been addressed. As mentioned in PART III Emotional Wellbeing, we can create stories and beliefs that skew our world view to keep us safe from overwhelming emotional experiences or trauma. Emotional pain is deemed, by the brain, as unsafe and so will keep you safe by creating a different narrative to follow. It is unlocking these deeper beliefs that is the key to you liberation.

Every single thought, word and deed has brought you to your current reality. Now if you are not happy with your life and I mean every part, stop tolerating or compromising on what you know deep down doesn't feel good and what you don't want. Ask yourself what you do want? Open your heart, unlock the chains and admit to yourself in your wildest dreams, what would set your soul on fire and make your heart sing?

Then it is your choice what to do next. You can choose to be a victim or victor in your life experience. You choose whether to step up or step back. I have spoken to hundreds if not thousands of people and there are some who are not willing to accept they have a choice and that is ok. For some that are not ready to deal with that reality, the truth can be too jarring or painful that they recoil to the safety of their own mind. This isn't a judgement, just an observation. Being unwilling to accept there is a choice either because the alternative is too painful to bear or that you have to take responsibility for it will keep you stuck.

Look at where your life is right now. What are you committed to? Does it align with how you want your life to be? Where are you happy? Where are you unhappy? If you have not achieved what you said, what are you making important right now? Look at where you are blaming other people, situations or circumstances for your predicament. This is where you begin.

What are you doing more of that that doesn't serve you?

What are you doing less of that lights you up?

This isn't about creating more commitments. It is about streamlining and letting go of what you have committed to that you do not want and creating commitments that you do.

What if you simply decided to do LESS and be MORE? Doing less more efficiently?

Commitment doesn't sound exciting and yet it's the quality and component of any transformation that turns a potential into possibility, possibility into probability and probability into certainty. Without this consider that the opposite is true, that is, no commitment means no certainty. No certainty means a lack of predication which the brain deems unsafe.

Commitments aren't just a statement of what you hope might happen, they are a true decision supported by clear, exact and precise processes and parameters that make it more certain that the decision holds up more in challenging or stressful times. Don't be vague. To 'eat healthier' for example, is a vague statement. Think of your commitment as a precise declaration such as eat 5 portions of vegetables per day.

Consider the length of your commitment and what terms you place on them to create the best possible process to follow for you to maintain.

Setting a commitment with clear terms of how it will be applied to your life will make it easier to follow.

Don't create something too extreme that it becomes a chore. Start from where you are and stretch yourself as far as "I can and will do this" will be for you. It is not about the size of the commitment but seeing it through. Your commitments are personal to you. Forget about the results, focus on the processes, the daily steps. Your process leads to success.

TASK - Make more skilful Commitments

Make a list of commitments you want to make. For example it could be for your health, happiness, purpose, appearance, fitness, nutrition, finances, business/career, adventure, etc. For each commitment you have created, list why they are important to you and what you believe the consequences are of not fulfilling that commitment. Be as clear and specific as possible.

Use the following template:

[COMMITMENT] because [REASON IMPORTANT]. I believe that this commitment will serve me [HOW IT SERVES] and that by NOT upholding the commitment the cost to me will be [CONSEQUENCE]

Don't make them too extreme. Remember, start where you are at and stretch yourself as far as "I can and will do this" will be for you. Next create a clear and definite 'until and unless' statement of what constitutes fully meeting the commitment.

From the commitments you have created above, make it clear when the commitment will finish and what exceptions there may be e.g. going to bed at 10:30pm UNLESS I am out for a special occasion.

[COMMITMENT] until [DATE / GOAL] unless [EXCEPTION]

Remember it's not about the size of the commitment you make, but one that you will see through to the end.

Your commitments are for you, nobody else. Commit to the success of the process, the steps you take each day to honour your commitment.

| 43 |

Raise Your Standards

Protecting your health and wellbeing comes from setting your own life stall out. Having the courage to live it how you want to live it. You will likely upset people, they will be triggered and they may even attack you verbally, bring you down or call you crazy. You have become a mirror and they do not like the reflection.

What anyone else says or does has nothing to do with you. People often attack when they are unhappy about something, In this case, that could be your decision to raise your game. You cannot make anyone feel a certain way, how they allow it to resonate and affect them is on them and it's up to them to deal with that.

It happened to me when I changed careers 11 years ago.

It's easy to plod on in life and wonder why nothing changes. But we cannot solve a problem with the same mindset that created it. Something has to change.

Expecting a different result whilst doing the same things doesn't make sense and yet we can get caught up in that same routine unless we bring awareness to it. By challenging the thoughts and beliefs that don't serve you, you get to take responsibility for where you are right now and take a different action that will move you towards what you desire. But you have to do the work. It isn't handed to you on a plate. It's up to you what you no longer tolerate.

Glory comes to those who not only dare to begin, but keep moving forwards, who commit to creating a meaningful life for themselves and nobody else.

It takes effort. It is likely that you will feel discomfort, which requires an identity shift and when that happens you will feel resistance. You will have old scripts and beliefs rise up to keep you where you are; uncomfortable feelings and emotions that can derail you if you let them.

You will always go out of your way to prove those beliefs true unless you challenge them, feel into them and choose differently. When you do choose differently, you get to remind yourself of WHY this is important to you.

Health is the only thing we truly own and yet so many take it for granted. But when you don't make time for health, somewhere along the line you WILL make time for illness.

If you are not achieving what you want right now it's time for some brutal self-honesty. To look at your core values (you do know what they are right?) to look at what you stand for and against and push through the discomfort. You will likely have emotional attachments to situations and circumstances. You get to bring awareness to the feelings you have and with those feelings, no matter how uncomfortable they are, let them go. Removing the baggage holding you back is the key to moving forward.

It's time to raise your standards. To set boundaries to protect your time and energy... and sometimes sanity!

Ask yourself right now. Put the book down and write down the answers to the following questions:

What standards do you set?

What are you compromising on?

What boundaries do you have?

You will likely feel uncomfortable, and that is where the answers lie. You get to ask the difficult questions of yourself.

There is no 'trying' your best. That gives you a reason to let yourself off the hook. You either commit or you don't. You choose!

When you raise your standards you create non-negotiable agreements with yourself, you raise the bar. You set the standard you DO NOT compromise on!

Remember, check in with yourself and challenge your beliefs, you will always get what you commit to.

From there you simply do not let them slip. Write them down, cast them in stone. Make a point of reminding yourself of these agreements every day. Reflect to see if you have lived up to your own agreements. If you do 'slip' then that's where you start to do the work. That's when you do the hard yards. That's when you question and challenge your beliefs. That's when you step up and feel into the pain and face your adversity, your fear.

You will likely feel a mixture of emotions, usually stemming from what others might say. They do not live your life... YOU DO!

That's when you ask yourself without judgement, why did they slip? What could I have done differently? What can I put in place so I don't slip again?

You owe it to yourself to raise your standards.

Remember, health isn't just about exercise, you cannot out train a bad diet, and calorie restriction isn't what health is, that is a small part of it. I want to help you to bulletproof your health, physically, mentally, emotionally and spiritually.

So how are you living right now? Are you plodding along? Are you blaming and avoiding? Are you just existing, surviving day to day? Is that how you want to live? Existing? Or do you want to thrive? Take action out of faith by taking the steps and doing the work.

Are you removing what doesn't make you happy to make room for what does?

"If you keep avoiding what's difficult in life, you will keep leading a difficult life. There is no growth in comfort. Have faith and believe in yourself"

- DEAN COULSON

Are you taking responsibility for your life?

When you do you will go from 'survive' to 'THRIVE!'

Task: Create a list of impeccable agreements.

Create a list of agreements that you live up to and do not compromise on. Use the following areas of your live as a guide:

Body

Balance

Being

Business

Buzz

(You can find a detailed description of these 5 areas under the 'What is health anyway' chapter in PART I)

Raising your standard is not in the saying, it's in the doing. It's always about showing not telling, doing the work, taking the steps.

It's not in the wishing, it's in the willing, being willing to step up and do whatever it takes; the discipline to show up consistently, day after day, week after week.

So who are you being? What do you believe about yourself? Be honest. Look in that mirror and ask the question. Find out who you are, your identity, how you show up in the world. What are you identifying with? Who are you identifying as?

What are your current standards you are living by? Do they serve you?

Challenge the limiting beliefs. Are they true? What evidence do you have to validate that belief? Who would you be if those limiting beliefs did not exist?

Remember your effulgence is in the action you take. It WILL be uncomfortable, but you know this already. You get to choose the life you lead.

Drop the should have, would have, could have and change it to I must, I will, I am and see what happens.

| 44 |

How to Set Your Day up to Win

Most of your reality is not a given. It is shaped by your expectations, beliefs and thoughts you have formed about it, some of them from way back in childhood. These beliefs and expectations form part of your daily habits. So many can be counterproductive, however you can bring awareness to this reality and consciously reframe those habits and thought patterns into positive habits that will transform and empower your life significantly.

The most common trait of highly successful people is the recognition of the power they have in co-creating their reality through changing the way they think, believe or expect their reality to be. One of the most effective ways of changing our belief patterns is through practising and maintaining daily rituals.

I am being deliberate in using the word ritual over routine and here's why...

A routine is simply an action that needs to be done, while a ritual usually has the connotation of being done with a sense of purpose or meaningfulness.

By applying meaningfulness to and being mindful during a routine, it can become a ritual. The ritual makes the routine more of a subjective experience rather than simply a task to be completed. Bringing awareness and fully experiencing what you are doing can change its meaning. For example, creating space to eat healthily could involve nourishing your body, focusing on the taste and texture, taking your time and being conscious of how you chew.

Creating a morning ritual or structure is essential for you taking control of your day. It prepares your mind, body and spirit in a positive manner and shifts your focus onto what you can achieve and how you can achieve it. Your energy flows where your focus goes, so by creating positive daily rituals your energy flows into what you do want, not what you don't.

Do you wake up in the morning and dread the day ahead, especially on a Monday?

If you do, then it is in your power to change it. Take a look at yourself in the mirror. It's time for some brutally honest self-reflection. Are you happy in every area of your life? Ask yourself that question and see where your energy goes. If it goes up you are on the right track, if your energy goes down or it feels heavy then there are things to address. If you don't address it the universe will bring it around again until you do. No amount of avoidance will help you move forwards.

If you aren't happy, stop lying to yourself, drop the validations and justifications and start taking the steps to get your body, mind and spirit in alignment. Look at your thoughts, words and actions, are they congruent? Do they line up? Or are you saying one thing and doing something else?

Ask yourself the following questions...

"What do I value in my LIFE the most?"

"What am I willing to give up that does not serve me right now?"

"Am I taking the steps towards my goals every day?"

"How do I know if I am meeting my values and agreements that I have made to myself?"

"Is my behaviour congruent with my values and goals?"

Once what you are thinking, saying and doing are in alignment you will achieve your goals. So now you get to check whether you are. Be clear in what you want to achieve and WHY you want to achieve it. Write down your goals in important areas of your life.

Creating Rituals

Let's be clear, if you don't have at least 15 minutes to work on yourself every morning then you are not in control of your life. You must be in control your time. So either you are allowing others to dictate your time and energy or you are setting incorrect priorities. It's easy to get up 15 minutes earlier if that's what it takes to move forward.

Morning rituals give a structure enabling you to take control, so life happens for you NOT to you.

By 'priming' yourself you are preparing yourself to win. Be ruthless with your time, energy and confidence.

Here are examples of things you can consider adding to your morning ritual. Be mindful of what feels good for you. Although these are entirely optional, I will recommend what I consider important to add to help you. If you find yourself avoiding certain things (e.g. meditation) ask yourself why? So many people turn to physical exercise and forget the one thing that holds everything together, the brain. Mental training is just as important and meditation is perfect for brain training. Just as allowing yourself to fully feel your emotions (even the painful ones).

Make sure you cover all four elements of health with your rituals too; they all work in synergy to help you.

Morning Ritual Ideas

- Hydrate (e.g. 500ml filtered water + lemon)
- Meditation
- Diaphragmatic breathing (e.g. in through nose, out through the mouth, 4 seconds in, 4 seconds pause, 4 seconds out, 4 seconds pause)
- Mobility drill / stretching / foam rolling / yoga
- Exercise / moving with purpose
- Gratitude journal (gratitude and appreciation. What 3 things are you grateful for, who/what do you appreciate)
- Writing down your goals (write down your goals to remind yourself of what you want to achieve and why you do what you do)
- Eat a healthy breakfast mindfully (protein and fat based is a great option)
- Watch a TED talk to inspire you.
- Visualisation (see in your minds eye how you want your day to go)
- Listen to a podcast (Who inspires you and energises you?)
- Listen to uplifting music (create energy / mood playlists)
- Watch comedy (need a lift, watch your favourite shows/comedians on you tube)
- Read something inspirational (e.g. quotes or books)
- Be present in the moment – practise the power of now (bring awareness to everything around you, focus on the moment. This can be done with focused breathing too)
- Walking in nature
- Protein Smoothie
- Learn a language
- Some form of brain training

- Asking questions to bring awareness to your thoughts and beliefs.
- Journaling

Focus on activities that empower you. Ask the question, "If today was the last day of my life, would I be happy with what I'm about to do?" If the answer was "no", change it, life is way too short. Simple to say, harder to do, but it is doable.

Create 3 options with 3 different time frames. That way you can avoid the all or nothing approach and always have an option to prime your day. Consider Option A as the ritual you do when you have plenty of time, B less time and C if you are short on time. That way all your bases are covered. You set the rules, just make sure that they empower you to set up your day to win.

When considering your activities be very strict with your time, assign minutes to each task and stick to them, that way you know which option you will be doing, A, B or C.

Here are some examples that you can consider. Don't over think it. Adjust your available timings for your lifestyle.

Option A (45+ minutes)

- Hydrate Drink 500 ml water & lemon (1 min)
- Meditation (20 min)
- Write your goals (5 min)
- Journaling (10 min)
- Mobilise / stretch / roll / yoga (10 mins)
- Exercise with uplifting music 2 for 1! (60 minutes)
- Breakfast (15min)

121 minutes

Option B (30-45 minutes)

- Hydrate Drink 500 ml water & lemon (1 min)
- Meditation (10 min)
- Write your goals (5 min)
- Journaling (5 min)
- Exercise with uplifting music 2 for 1 (10 minutes)
- Breakfast (10 min)

41 minutes

Option C (15-30 minutes)

- Hydrate Drink 500 ml water & lemon (1 min)
- Diaphragmatic box breathing (5 min), focus on the breath.
- Write your goals (5 min)
- Mobilise / stretch / roll / yoga (5 mins)
- Breakfast smoothie (5 min)

21 minutes

These are not hard and fast but are designed to help you create a 'peak state' where you feel energised and invigorated to win your day.

Bookending your day

This modern world affords so much opportunity, but can court chaos and stress if we allow it. Trying to fit in so much in, leads to long, extended days and insufficient sleep. Restorative rest and recovery are imperative for your health.

Your next day starts the night before. How you wind down (or not) before bed has an impact on how your next day will go. Nourishing your body with good food and preparing your body for restful sleep is imperative (see the chapter 'I can't get no sleep' for more information) to prime you for the following morning to hit the ground running. Once you create a wind down ritual stick to it. Your circadian rhythm loves structure and routine.

Also clear your head. We often carry the stresses of the day into the evening and don't allow ourselves to unwind.

Two things can and will help with this if you are consistent; counting your wins and journaling.

Counting your wins

Allow yourself to appreciate what you have achieved in your day. Count three wins, no matter how big or small for that day, allow your mind to end the day in a positive frame. It could be as simple as getting out of bed, or reading a book or bigger wins like completing a course or signing up a new client. Writing them down in a journal creates space in a busy mind.

Journaling

Most of us live way too much in our heads which can frequently lead to stress and overwhelm. When we don't allow ourselves to slow down, journaling allows us to get some of what is in our heads onto paper.

Over time with so much going on, our brains develop patterns of habitual behaviours which we just fall into; that autopilot feeling, without really challenging whether they serve us.

Journaling allows you to explore new ideas and new possibilities and identify problems and challenges; highlighting what is keeping you stuck and what to do about it.

By being disciplined, journaling starts bypassing the surface level stuff you cannot get past and allows a deeper exploration of new possibilities and challenging your beliefs.

The action of journaling and just writing without thought allows you to write from the heart without your conscious filters, to get out what has been festering. Write with no thought, just allow it to flow. Just start writing!

Remember we live too much in our heads, creating realities that do not serve us. Daily journaling allows you to clear that out and write from the heart.

The simplest form of journaling is introducing the concept of AM and PM prompts.

Use simple questions at the start and end of each day to direct your focus. Here are some examples...

AM Journaling Prompts

Three things I'm grateful for... This question takes you from a state of expectation to appreciation. Expectation is trying to control your external world. Appreciation allows you to focus on your internal world.

Come up with new answers every day. Look at it as new thinking, NOT remembering. If you feel stuck, ask yourself why you were grateful for what you wrote yesterday and allow yourself to look deeper.

Three priorities for the day ahead... This allows you a bit of focus, which builds confidence. E.g. complete my journaling, catch up with a friend, read a book for 20 minutes.

PM Journaling Prompts

What did I learn today? E.g. I learned box breathing

Who did I positively impact?

These questions are part of our human needs, growth and contribution that we often forget about. This adds to our fulfilment and sense of peace and harmony.

Remember these questions are about awareness, so don't be too hard on yourself. Let go of any expectation you may have. The process shines a light on what to focus on to make more of an effort with.

Write these prompts in your journal along with your 3 wins each evening.

We have a negativity bias to keep us safe, but often these get over developed. Asking ourselves better questions allows us to see things differently.

We often focus on what we don't want, however, asking better questions of ourselves allows us to focus on what we do want. When we ask better quality questions we get better quality answers.

So set some time with no distractions to journal.

A lot of stress in life is when we see a situation we believe without seeing any other perspective. Allow yourself to be open to any and all possibilities and your mind will expand.

| 45 |

Warrior Practices

Being a martial artist I trained to defend myself and my family from harm. But it was more than that. Martial arts for me was not just physical but meta-physical; it is a set of values and morals to live by, the martial way. Courtesy, integrity, perseverance and self-control (the tenets of my first martial art, Jintian Do). It is also about discipline, resilience, tenacity and repetition or being consistent.

I always looked to fight my way out of situations, but I don't mean physically, although I would if I had to. I mean mentally and emotionally. That's when I realised, it's not about the fight but the surrender, letting go of things that no longer (or never) served me. That's not to say you don't stand up for what you believe in, but you don't keep doing things that are out of balance with who you are.

I created the '12 rounds' Warrior Practices as a way to guide you to build an indomitable spirit; to build courage through awareness, take personal responsibility and action. Remember the definition of a warrior is having the courage to face one's self. To challenge the thoughts and beliefs you hold by going inside. Make no mistake it is the most challenging thing you will ever do, but also the most rewarding. Your liberation comes from having the courage to face and let go of your fears.

| 46 |

The 12 Rounds

Round 1: The Warrior Creed

Every martial artist fights for something. They stand for a set of moral values; the way of the warrior; how they conduct themselves in the face of adversity. It all starts with self-protection against the self, not just physically but psychologically, turning in to face the difficult areas in their life, where only the brave choose to go. Whether stepping into the arena or in life, choosing into areas of 'difficult / difficult', where they feel fear and still choose to master each area (Physically, emotionally, mentally and spiritually) knowing that it will lead to success. Confidence comes from clarity. Clarity comes from simplicity. Simplicity comes from knowing. A warrior knows who they are and what to do and take action to gain self-sovereignty over themselves.

Warrior Practice: There is no grow in comfort. Explore the concept of 'high altitude' living. To master yourself, you must first master your palate; what you ingest, what you take in through the senses (food, gossip, tv, news, radio). Master your senses and everything else falls into line. Refuse to settle. Explore and write down all the difficult situations you are avoiding. Admit them to yourself and face them one by one to gain power. Find where the discomfort lies and transmute it into positive energy.

Round 2: What Will You Fight For?

A fighter knows what he is fighting for. Most people go through life reacting to what it throws at them, feeling as if they're constantly fighting, but with no sense of purpose. They are not clear on who they are and what they stand for. Constantly reacting to life instead of being proactive, being controlled instead of taking control. When you don't stand for something, you fall for everything.

Warrior Practice - Write down a list of statements that you believe in and make a list of your values – such as trust, success, and courage. Find 3 value words that resonate with you and explain why. Use them as a compass in every decision you make.

Round 3: Pick Your Shots

A fighter doesn't waste energy throwing random punches and kicks; they conserve their energy and make the strikes count. In life, it's important to know not just what you want but why you want it. Just doing things randomly without purpose will not get you where you want to be or the happiness you crave. Be specific, clear and precise about what you do want with laser beam focus.

Warrior Practice: What does your perfect day look like? What would you be doing? Who would you be with? Where would you live? What can you do today to start taking steps towards that life?

Round 4: Know Your Opponent

A fighter gets to know their opponent before stepping into the arena. The word warrior literally translates to one with the courage to face themselves. You have all the answers, you just don't realise. It is often easier to look externally, but that search will be fruitless. In life your biggest opponent is yourself, because you go into 'threat' mode. Triune brain theory divides the brain into human, animal and reptile. When the brain has no way of predicting and responding to a situation safely, it relies on the animal part of our brain which deals with survival and gets stuck in 'fight or flight' mode.

Warrior Practice: Identify and understand the threats in your life. What stresses you out? What are the triggers? Where do you feel unsafe? Where do you keep going round in circles? Plan responses and how you react to these stresses to change your path. Face each one down, feel into every reaction and sensation and let them go.

Round 5: Finding Balance

A fighter can't fight properly if they're off balance; they will go down the first time they're hit. Many people live in survival mode and are on their way to adrenal burnout and chronic fatigue. They push and push for what they think is the most important thing to them, usually career success, only to realise once they reach it, that it was least important of all. Their lives suddenly feel hollow and incomplete. They feel out of alignment with themselves and with those they hold most dear.

Warrior Practice: Allow yourself time for relaxation, whatever works for you; meditation, yoga, walking, reading or getting out in nature. Create space for yourself daily. Just stop and be you.

Round 6: Trust Your Guard

A fighter never forgets to keep their guard up to protect themselves from being hit. Having a strong guard is having a strong sense of self. So when life throws you punches, as it often does, remember your values and ask yourself how can I react and respond differently? You always have a choice. If you react in a negative way to a situation or circumstance, even if it is not directed at you, then that becomes your teacher. Something inside you resonates and it is up to you to turn inside and find out what it is.

Warrior Practice: Trust your values, and believe in what you stand for. Develop certainty in your beliefs. Challenge them to see if they stand up. Do what you said you would. Take small steps every day to create momentum towards what you said you would do.

Round 7: Find Your Fighting Style

Each fighter has their own unique fighting style. Many of our struggles take place because we are trying to live up to other people's definitions of us. Everyone from parents to teachers tries to mould us into a version that they think is best. The trouble is, this sticks on the hard drive (our mind) from a young age and can shape our view of the world. We have to shed this image and define ourselves. Challenge our stories, scripts and beliefs and find out what we stand for and against.

Warrior Practice: Think again about your values, and answer the following question for each one. "If I was living this value, I would be feeling / doing / saying..."

Round 8: Master Your Defence

A fighter has a defence for every shot that's likely to be thrown at them and adapts accordingly. Be ready with an offence to face threats such as other people's judgement, expectation, perfectionism, opinions, and comparison to others. Defining and believing in your core values will help you to realign with who you are and keep your attention to who you are.

Warrior Practice: Identify the threat you're feeling and then change the angle. Practise calm breathing; change your state by exercising or listening to music that inspires and motivates you, allowing you to tune into the true version of yourself. Change the arena and step into your power.

Round 9: Stop the Trash Talk

Fighters always use an element of trash talk with each other before stepping into the arena to mentally wear their opponent down. We often 'trash talk' ourselves, and it stops us winning. We put ourselves down far too often, wasting vital time and energy. Our energy flows where our focus goes. You can think of this as A.N.T.s – Automatic Negative Thoughts. Be aware of how you think, what you say and what you do as a result of that thought.

Warrior Practice: When you hear that negative voice in your head, ask, "What are you saying about yourself? Is that story true? Who would I be without that story?" Challenge every thought that prevents you from being the real you. Look for evidence.

Round 10: Keep Your Guard Up

A fighter never walks into their opponent's shots unprepared. They visualise how the fight will go in their favour. Every move and counter is rehearsed and mentally thought out. Failure does not even enter their minds. Consider how to set up your day and influence your environment to your advantage. What could you do first thing in the morning to get the day off to a good start? For some it might be as simple as a quiet cuppa alone before the rest of the family wake up or doing some exercise or meditating. Control your day before the day controls you.

Warrior Practice: Create a morning and evening ritual that puts you in control. Using the concept of 'No gaps', make sure you leave no stone unturned in filling your day how you want it to be. If you don't plan your time for what you want to do and achieve, someone else will fill the gap for you. Creating rituals allows you to take back control of you, your energy and time.

Round 11: Who's In Your Corner?

No fighter would ever step into the arena without a strong team to support them. So who is in your corner to support and encourage you? Equally, are you turning to people who aren't really helping, bringing you down or criticising? Make sure that you have people around you who support you and have your best interests at heart. Remember, if you are accepting other people's opinions of you over your own opinion of yourself, then they are not someone to be around or listened to.

Warrior Practice: Think about the 5 people you spend most time with and ask yourself, "Do they support me or criticise me? Do they help or hinder me?" Make sure that you only spend time with people who inspire you. We often do things to makes others feel better to the detriment of our own happiness. Ask yourself why that is important and see what comes up. You always come first... ALWAYS!

Round 12: Shadow Boxing

A fighter shadow boxes every day to practise their attack and defence combinations. To master a technique requires Attention, Intention & Repetition (A.I.R.). To create real lasting transformation, focus the brain, keep your attention on what is important and what you want to achieve. Be mindful of any distractions and remove then. KEEP YOUR FOCUS. Remind yourself of what you said you wanted and why it is important to you. Repeat the actions required enough times for them to become a habit.

Warrior Practice: Work on yourself first every day, set up rituals that you can practice daily. Define your strategies for success. Create the discipline to perform your rituals every day. Be consistent, persistent and frequent to achieve success.

| 47 |

A Call to Arms!

Are you living and loving your life to the full right now?

Are you addressing every part of the health paradigm in this book?

Are you being fully present or have you noticed how much time you spend anchored in the past or projected into the future? Influenced by past conditioning, stories and beliefs, those societal mores and cultural bias that permeate every part of your life.

Are you being who you were expected to be, not who you wanted to be?

Are you being distracted by random thoughts that take you off track, off balance and away from your calm centre; away from the life you said you wanted.

Thoughts flow from the past or into the future. They are influenced by experiences stored in the mind. The thing is, are you of your own mind or influenced by someone elses?

When you make a commitment to be in the present moment you allow your heart to open and sing, trusting your intuition to help guide you. To keep you in the immersive experience of committing to being fully present. But so many people do not trust themselves. They allow self-doubt to control their lives.

Ask yourself how much of your life was YOUR idea?

Have you ever considered whose life you are really leading?

How much of you was inherent or inherited?

Who were you before you became what the world told you to be?

Are you really in control?

When will you release yourself from those mind forged manacles?

When will you start living your life by design NOT by default?

When will you start using your powerful imagination instead of your indoctrination?

We have become more and more disconnected from our bodies; no longer in tune with the way our bodies feel or the way our minds think.

Every day we validate our choices. How often have you heard yourself think or say the following...

"This food bloats me but I am still going to eat it"

"It's ok to have a glass of wine every night, it's just the one"

"I'm a night owl, I don't need that much sleep"

"I can't be bothered to exercise this week, I will start back on Monday"

Just to make it clear, disease is not a mystery. It is a result of the choices we make, every single day.

The bill always becomes due.

So what are you validating?

You know when your spark is ignited or extinguished. YOU KNOW!

You know if you are surviving or THRIVING in your life!

When you allow yourself to be fully present you create a commitment to yourself to BE you.

Your intuition knows the answer. Stop thinking and start feeling. Get out of your head and open your heart. Inner certainty comes from trusting in yourself and having the faith that everything will be ok.

Will you find the courage to ignite your spark and work from a place of knowing and certainty in who you really are?

Health is multifaceted, there is no one thing. It is always a combination of things that can change everything for you and allow you to THRIVE!

What to do next?

Before you dive in head first and try and do all the things in this book at once, STOP!

I am sure you have tried many times before with limited success. Stop looking for the instant gratification. If you are not thriving in your life, ask yourself how long have you been feeling like that? It will take time to undo years of poor health choices. This is when you choose to take back control and realise health isn't a sometime thing, it's an ALL time thing.

It's time to follow a holistic approach to your health. Focus on mind, body and spirit. Your physical, mental, emotional and spiritual wellbeing work synergistically; they all impact each other. You cannot consider one without the other.

The foundations of health are simple.

Consider the following:

Optimising circadian rhythm

Optimal sleep

Stress reduction

Eating patterns.

Hydration

Physical activity (not just exercise)

Emotional wellbeing

Gratitude

Supplementation (if required)

Environment

Once these are established, symptoms will improve. If not, consider what else could be impacting your health.

Is there a disease present? What other symptoms are presenting? Looking at the whole picture is vital and as important as diet is, it isn't the be all and end all of health, it's just another piece of the jigsaw.

Assess where you are in your life right now with regards to your physical, mental, emotional and spiritual health. What do you feel you need to improve?

Score each section above on a scale between 1 and 5 (1 being the lowest, 5 meaning you are thriving). Pick one or two things from the areas where you have scored lowest and integrate them into your daily rituals for at least seven days. Do not overwhelm yourself.

Set your day up to win by creating morning and evening rituals based on what you want to improve. Look at each part of the book for what you can do to build those rituals.

Set commitments that stretch you a little bit. If you haven't set your commitments over each area of health, go back to the task at the end of the commitments chapter and do the work.

Every day, take small steps consistently towards your commitments. Do you feel motivated? If not, why not. Bring awareness to your thoughts and feelings in that moment? Do you feel safe? Challenge those thoughts to see if they are really true, be aware of your feelings around them and create time to sit with them and clear them.

The power is in the process, the steps you take every day, consistently, persistently and frequently and letting go of expectation.

It's important to understand what is common in this world is NOT normal. You have the ability to respond differently based on what is true for you.

Stop making things complicated. The gift is in the simplicity. If you are making life complicated you have unconscious self-limiting beliefs and stories making it complicated to keep you safe. As crazy as that sounds if you have labelled something wrongly or unsafe maybe due to some past overwhelming emotional experience or trauma, your ego will go out of its way to keep you safe from it. However, if you put it there, you can remove it and replace it with a better story. You can create a new reality any time you choose.

Pain is the root cause of behaviour. We will always move away from pain as it is part of our survival response. We understand physical pain, however sometimes the threat comes from within, our overwhelming emotional trauma that remains raw and unresolved. Emotional pain sucks and our brain protects us accordingly. It can and often does influence our choices. We are at times literally out of our minds. Often we attack and lash out from projected pain we harbour within. We have to be aware of how we react and what we are avoiding and in that moment we have the choice to be brave, to pause, feel and respond differently. When we hear it, see it, feel it, meet it, love it, it releases. Pausing is powerful, it is the first step to self-mastery and taking back control of your life.

Replace the stories that hold you back, challenge them, question them and feel into them. Let that energy go, recoup the effulgence and take that power back. Ask yourself what am I trusting in right now? Is it serving me? Is it taking me forwards or holding me back? CHALLENGE EVERYTHING!!! Find your alignment, check in with yourself often. Do your thoughts, words and actions align with your values, what you stand for and against? If not feel into those beliefs, rewire and release them.

To move from surviving to thriving requires courage, it requires you to step out from the shadows, to stand up for what you believe in, to be aware of how you think and feel, take responsibility for your own life and take action.

Now it's time to THRIVE!

REFERENCES

Lost history of medicine: http://www.mnwelldir.org/docs/terrain/lost_history_of_medicine.htm

Physiology, Cortisol: https://www.ncbi.nlm.nih.gov/books/NBK538239/

The effects of chronic stress on health: new insights into the molecular mechanisms of brain–body communication: https://www.ncbi.nlm.nih.gov/pmc/articles/PMC5137920/

The protective role of exercise on stress system dysregulation and co-morbidities: https://pubmed.ncbi.nlm.nih.gov/17148741/

Stress, Food, and Inflammation: Psychoneuroimmunology and Nutrition at the Cutting Edge: https://www.ncbi.nlm.nih.gov/pmc/articles/PMC2868080/

Gut microbiome diversity is associated with sleep physiology in humans https://pubmed.ncbi.nlm.nih.gov/31589627/

Gut microbiome composition and diversity are related to human personality traits https://www.sciencedirect.com/science/article/pii/S2452231719300181

Role of the gut microbiota in nutrition and health https://www.bmj.com/content/361/bmj.k2179

Chronic Sleep Disruption Alters Gut Microbiota, Induces Systemic and Adipose Tissue Inflammation and Insulin Resistance in Mice https://www.nature.com/articles/srep35405?fbclid=IwAR1Dr9polx-l1qz2Zao_kK3Hl2pxcI_Gt-2RScdo7nVjBJnSTeqLYC0Ljqg

The awakening response and blood glucose levels: https://pubmed.ncbi.nlm.nih.gov/10201642/

Importance of maintaining a low omega–6/omega–3 ratio for reducing inflammation https://www.ncbi.nlm.nih.gov/pmc/articles/PMC6269634/

An Increase in the Omega-6/Omega-3 Fatty Acid Ratio Increases the Risk for Obesity https://www.ncbi.nlm.nih.gov/pmc/articles/PMC4808858/

Effect of a high-protein breakfast on the postprandial ghrelin response. https://pubmed.ncbi.nlm.nih.gov/16469977/

Critical role for peptide YY in protein-mediated satiation and body-weight regulation. https://pubmed.ncbi.nlm.nih.gov/16950139/

A high-protein diet induces sustained reductions in appetite, ad libitum caloric intake, and body weight despite compensatory changes in diurnal plasma leptin and ghrelin concentrations https://pubmed.ncbi.nlm.nih.gov/16002798/

The effects of consuming frequent, higher protein meals on appetite and satiety during weight loss in overweight/obese men https://pubmed.ncbi.nlm.nih.gov/20847729/

The effects of high protein diets on thermogenesis, satiety and weight loss: a critical review https://pubmed.ncbi.nlm.nih.gov/15466943/

Gluconeogenesis and energy expenditure after a high-protein, carbohydrate-free diet https://pubmed.ncbi.nlm.nih.gov/19640952/

Energy expenditure and protein requirements after traumatic injury
https://pubmed.ncbi.nlm.nih.gov/16998142/

Dietary protein to maximize resistance training: a review and examination of protein spread and change theories
https://pubmed.ncbi.nlm.nih.gov/22958314/

The effects of protein supplements on muscle mass, strength, and aerobic and anaerobic power in healthy adults: a systematic review
https://pubmed.ncbi.nlm.nih.gov/25169440/

The Triune Brain (2016), Dahlitz, M https://www.thescienceofpsychotherapy.com/the-triune-brain/

Meditation, Process and effects: https://www.ncbi.nlm.nih.gov/pmc/articles/PMC4895748/

The food additive-free diet in the treatment of behaviour disorders
https://pubmed.ncbi.nlm.nih.gov/3949989/

Sleep is vital to associating emotion with memory https://www.sciencedaily.com/releases/2021/02/210222164216.htm

Emotional Wellbeing

Special thanks to Tim Neale and Tracy Hamilton from Rise and Shine for allowing me to reproduce their human needs framework diagram.

ACKNOWLEDGEMENTS

To the people who have helped me get to where I am today, who have been there for me, given me help, support and had faith in me, I just wanted to say thank you.

Joy Coulson. My soul mate. Thank you for your unwavering belief in me and for standing shoulder to shoulder with me in the dark times and the good times. You inspire me every single day and I am in awe of your energy and kind spirit. I have loved you long before I even met you x.

Sam Coulson. My miracle, who we were told was an impossibility. You changed my life for the better and you fill my heart with joy. My love for you knows no bounds, I am proud to be your Deeds. Love you buddy x.

John & Dot Coulson. For being the best parents I could wish for, thank you for believing in me and for having faith in me, you have always been there when I needed you.

Geoff Thompson. Your teachings and friendship have literally changed my life. You opened my eyes to what was really possible and why I was placed here on this planet. I will be eternally grateful to you for that.

Michael Heppell. For believing in me and seeing the shining light I often don't see and encouraging me to write this boooook! You are simply brilliant!

Dax Moy. For your mad ramblings, coaching and friendship. My life is better because you have been in it. At times you have challenged every fibre of my being and got me to question who I really am. Your lessons have been profound and I appreciate every single one.

Cliff Wilde. Your generosity to share your knowledge on health allowed me to see way beyond the dogma and question my own beliefs to allow me to take my knowledge on health to a deeper level. You sir are a genius.

Tim Neale. For allowing me to find the missing piece of the health jigsaw I was searching for and finding my brother from another mother. Our life journeys are so similar it is startling. Thank you for you friendship and support.

Tracy Hamilton. Since we first met, your help, guidance and support has been invaluable. My awareness of self has expanded because you challenge me every week. You have always been there for me without judgement, holding space for me to just be so I could work things through. Thank you.

Mark Whitehand. The long haired, short haired Yorkshireman, you have gone beyond the call of duty so many times I have lost count. I know you only ever have my best interests at heart and have always gone the extra mile. An amazing coach and greater friend.

Dan Meredith. For one email that changed my perspective and reminded me that I will achieve my dreams no matter how long it takes. Your words resonated deeply and my mind returns to them frequently.

Bob Sykes. For allowing me to write about nutrition and health in the UK's largest martial arts magazine, Martial Arts Illustrated. It was a pleasure to be a part of a national institution that ran for many years. When I bought my first issue many years ago, I never ever considered being part of it.

Kenn Forrest. Our friendship has stood the test of time from being a wee nipper to the present day. I always value our conversations, the training and the laughs. It's an honour to call you a friend.

Diane Hull, Philippa Mathewson, Angela Beeston and Kevin Harvey (aka topgunners). For standing by me every step of the way to get this book over the line. I cannot express what your friendship means to me, but I suspect you already know

To everyone else I have crossed paths with on my life's journey and have had a positive and negative impact, thank you. Every single interaction has lead me to this point and make me who I am.

BIBLIOGRAPHY

I have a large library of books, too many books to reference here. But I would like to highlight some of them that have influenced the writing of this book.

Warrior by Geoff Thompson

Shapeshifter by Geoff Thompson

Why Zebras Don't Get Ulcers by Robert Sapolsky

Behave, the Best and Worst of Humans by Robert Sapolsky

In Search of the Miraculous by Orspenski

The Optimum Nutrition Bible by Patrick Holford

Natural Solutions to Infertility by Marilyn Glenville

Eat, Move & be healthy by Paul Chek.

Nutrition and Physical Degeneration by Weston A Price

How Not to Die by Michael Greger

Sick and Tired: Reclaim your inner terrain by Robert Young

The Terrain is Everything: Contextual factors that influence our health by Susan Stockton

Meet Your Happy Chemicals by Loretta Graziano Breuning

Parasite Rex by Carl Zimmer

Flip It by Michael Heppell

Breaking the Habit Of Being Yourself by Dr Joe Dispenza

Conversations With God by Neale Donald Walsch

Waking the Tiger: Healing trauma by Peter Levine

The Body Keeps the Score by Bessel Van Der Kolk

Unique Healing 2: A Guide for Eliminating Your "A-Z" Symptoms, Weight problems, illnesses and addictions by Donna Pessin

MY GIFT TO YOU

Every reader of THRIVE! will get access to bonuses to compliment this book – freebies and resources to help you implement what you learn from THRIVE!

If you would like more resources, ideas, videos, articles and a whole bunch of goodies the please visit www.theleanwarrior.com/thriveresources or use the QR code or the website below for access.

KEEP IN TOUCH

For information on the courses and programs I run as well as speaking engagements, masterclasses and events please go to www.theleanwarrior.com for more information.

I hope you have enjoyed learning about how to THRIVE! I wish you every success.

Need more help? Do you want to join me? Here's how:

- Join me on My Warrior Within program at www.theleanwarrior.com

- Work with me one to one.

- Download my podcasts

- Subscribe to my YouTube channel

Share your success stories with me from your experience with the book. I'd love to hear from you.

Email them to: success@theleanwarrior.com

To your success,

Dean Coulson

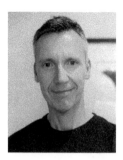

After been told he could never have kids and 2 failed IVF attempts, Dean embarked upon a path uncovering what true health meant to see if there was another way. It turned out there was, optimising health is so powerful, his son was conceived naturally. From that point Dean was curious what else was possible and discovered his true purpose. Empowering and inspiring others to be all that they are. Using a holistic approach to optimise what Dean see's as the 4 elements of health and well-being (physical, mental, emotional and spiritual), that allow us to thrive.

From IT consultant to gym owner and now a highly acclaimed performance lifestyle coach, Dean help's successful businessmen, entrepreneurs and CEO's who are stressed, anxious and feel burnt out, optimise their health and performance so that they can relax, feel happy and fulfilled and spend more time with their family. Showing men how to remove fears and express who they really are by giving them the tools and resources to thrive in all areas for their life.

Martial arts has been a huge part of his life for over 30 years and has studied a number of martial arts to black belt and has been inducted into the UK black belt martial arts hall of fame. He uses his experiences to provide a unique coaching experience to defend against your inner bully and overcome whatever life throws at you.

Lightning Source UK Ltd.
Milton Keynes UK
UKHW020650250721
387661UK00002B/2/J